Stage 3 Kidney Disease

Diet Cookbook for Seniors

Easy-to-Follow Nutritious Low Sodium, Low Phosphorus & Low Potassium Recipes for the Elderly to Manage Stage 3 CKD and Prevent Renal Failure

Cynthia P. Allison

Copyright © 2024 by Cynthia P. Allison

All rights reserved. No part of this publication may be reproduced, distributed, or transmitted in any form or by any means, including photocopying, recording, or other electronic or mechanical methods, without the prior written permission of the author, except in the case of brief quotations embodied in critical reviews and certain other noncommercial uses permitted by copyright law.

The recipes, information, and advice provided in this book are based on the author's research and experience. However, readers are encouraged to consult with healthcare professionals or qualified experts regarding their specific dietary needs, health conditions, or concerns.

The author and publisher disclaim responsibility for any adverse effects or consequences resulting from the use of the information presented in this book. The inclusion of brand names or links does not imply endorsement or association with the author.

Every effort has been made to ensure the accuracy of the information presented. Still, the author and publisher cannot be held responsible for errors or omissions, or any consequences arising from the use of the information contained herein.

About the Author

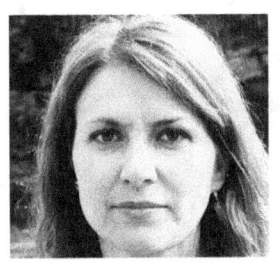Cynthia P. Allison, the creative force behind this insightful cookbook, is a Nutritionist and a seasoned writer with a passion for exploring the intersection of health and culinary arts. With a background in nutrition and a keen interest in a Healthy Kidney lifestyle, Cynthia has dedicated her profession and writing skills to empower individuals managing chronic kidney disease.

Her expertise goes beyond words on paper; Cynthia is committed to delivering practical solutions and inspiring a mindful approach to eating. Drawing from real-life experiences and a genuine commitment to well-being, she shares not only delicious recipes but a holistic perspective on achieving kidney health through the lens of the Renal Diet.

Cynthia P. Allison represents the amalgamation of knowledge, creativity, and a genuine desire to make a positive impact on the lives of her readers. Join Cynthia on this culinary journey, where health meets flavor, and discover the transformative power of the stage 4 Kidney Disease Diet Cookbook for Seniors.

Explore, savor, and thrive with Cynthia P. Allison.

Positive Affirmations for Seniors with Stage 3 Kidney Disease

"I embrace each day with gratitude and optimism, knowing that I am taking positive steps towards a healthier future".

Table of Contents

INTRODUCTION 9

1. UNDERSTANDING YOUR KIDNEY 13
   Kidney Function And Filtration 13
   How Kidney Mal-function Starts, the Progression of Kidney Disease 14

2. INTRODUCTION TO STAGE 3 KIDNEY DISEASE 15
   What is stage 3 CKD (Chronic kidney disease) 15
   Causes and risk factors of stage 3 CKD 15
   Implications of Stage 3 CKD on seniors 16
   Importance of Early Detection & Intervention 17
   Medical Diagnosis and Treatment 17
   Needs for dietary modifications in managing stage 3 CKD 18

3. DIETARY GUIDELINES FOR SENIORS ON STAGE 3 KIDNEY DISEASE 21
   Balancing electrolytes 21
   Balancing macronutrients 22
   Balancing Fluid Intake 23
   Protein requirements 24
   Vitamins and minerals crucial for seniors on stage 3 ckd 25
   Daily Nutrient Recommendation for Seniors on Stage 3 CKD 27

4. ESSENTIAL KITCHEN PRACTICES FOR SENIORS ON STAGE 3 CKD 29
   Basic Required Kitchen Tools 29
   Ingredients and Pantry Staples 30
   Ingredients Substitution 31
   Cooking Techniques Suitable for Seniors with Stage 3 Kidney Disease 32
   Tips on Reducing Nutrients on Every Day Meals 34
   Meal Planning and Portion Management 35
   Label-reading Techniques 37

5. KIDNEY-FRIENDLY RECIPES FOR SENIORS ON STAGE 3 KIDNEY DISEASE 39
BREAKFAST 39
   Veggie Omelette 39

Overnight Oats..40
Greek Yogurt Parfait..41
Avocado Toast...42
Breakfast Burrito...43
Quinoa Breakfast Bowl...44
Spinach and Feta Frittata Muffins...45
Berry Smoothie...46
Cottage Cheese Pancakes..47
Breakfast Bowl with Sweet Potatoes..48

LUNCH..51
Grilled Chicken Salad...51
Lentil Soup...52
Tuna Salad Wrap...53
Quinoa Salad with Roasted Vegetables...54
Turkey and Veggie Sandwich on Whole Wheat Bread....................................55
Vegetable Stir-Fry with Brown Rice...56
Chickpea Salad with Feta and Cucumber...57
Salmon and Avocado Sushi Bowl..58
Black Bean Quesadilla with Guacamole..59
Greek Salad with Grilled Shrimp..60

DINNER..63
Baked Salmon with Lemon and Herbs..63
Chicken Stir-Fry with Broccoli and Bell Peppers..64
Vegetable Curry with Tofu...65
Turkey Meatballs with Whole Wheat Pasta...66
Roasted Vegetable and Quinoa Stuffed Bell Peppers....................................67
Shrimp and Vegetable Skewers with Brown Rice..68
Eggplant Parmesan with Whole Wheat Spaghetti...69
Beef and Vegetable Stir-Fry with Cauliflower Rice..71
Lentil and Vegetable Soup..72

DESSERTS & SNACKS RECIPES...75
Fruit Salad with Honey-Lime Dressing..75
Dark Chocolate-Dipped Strawberries..76
Greek Yogurt with Fresh Berries and Almonds..77
Baked Apple Slices with Cinnamon...78

Homemade Trail Mix with Nuts, Seeds, and Dried Fruit...................................79
Cottage Cheese with Pineapple and Toasted Coconut..80
Rice Cake with Almond Butter..80
Greek Yogurt Bark with Mixed Nuts and Dark Chocolate Chips........................81
Baked Sweet Potato Chips with Sea Salt...82

SOUP & SALAD RECIPES..84
Minestrone Soup..84
Chicken Noodle Soup...85
Butternut Squash Soup..86
Greek Salad...88
Caesar Salad...89
Spinach Salad with Strawberries and Walnuts..90
Quinoa Salad...91
Caprese Salad...92

BEVERAGES...95
Cucumber Mint Cooler..95
Berry Blast Smoothie..96
Watermelon Limeade..97
Ginger Turmeric Tea...98
Green Tea Matcha Latte..99

6. KICK START YOUR JOURNEY TO HEALTHIER YOU..................................101
Unique Easy to follow 35 Day Meal Plans Tailored for seniors with stage 3 ckd..101
Detailed Comprehensive Grocery Shopping Lists for Convenience.............104
Proteins...104
Vegetables...104
Fruits...105
Grains..105
Legumes..105
Dairy and Alternatives..106
Nuts and Seeds..106
Herbs and Spices...106
Other...107
Foods to Eat and Avoid...108
Accurate Methods Of Using Gram/ounce..109

7. LIFESTYLE TIPS 111
Hydration, Supplements, Exercise, and Stress Management 111
Why Medical Check-ups 112
Dining Out Strategy 113

CONCLUSION 115

BONUS 119
Bonus 1: Free Email Consultation 119
Bonus 2: 25 Kidney Health Quiz Questions With Answers for Seniors With Stage 3 Kidney Disease 119

INTRODUCTION

Stage 3 Chronic Kidney Disease (CKD) is a silent killer that affects millions of people globally when it comes to health issues that seniors encounter. Known for a mild decline in kidney function, this stage requires aggressive therapy and close observation, especially in the older population.

The number of individuals in the United States alone believed to have chronic kidney disease (CKD) is around 37 million, according to the Centers for Disease Control and Prevention (CDC), many of whom are unaware that they have the illness. Moreover, CKD is a serious public health problem, according to the National Kidney Foundation, it affects 10% of people worldwide.

The concerning increase in risk factors linked to kidney disease, such as diabetes, hypertension, obesity, and cardiovascular disease, exacerbates this problem. These illnesses add to the rising prevalence of renal failure, which is the ninth-largest cause of mortality worldwide due to kidney disease.

Moreover, racial and ethnic minorities continue to have greater rates of renal disease and its consequences than other demographic groups, indicating persistent inequities in kidney health. Kidney disease also has a large financial cost burden, putting a heavy load on both people and healthcare systems due to treatment, dialysis, and transplantation expenditures.

To lessen the effects of kidney disease and improve the prognosis for those who are impacted, these figures highlight the critical need for increased awareness, preventative initiatives, and access to early diagnosis and treatment measures.

Consider your body as an intricately balanced apparatus, with every organ contributing significantly to its seamless functioning. This delicate equilibrium is upset for elderly patients with Stage 3 CKD because their kidneys are unable to adequately remove waste products and extra fluid from the circulation. Its effects go much beyond minor annoyance; there are serious implications for life expectancy and general health.

The function of nutrition presents itself as a ray of light in this hopeless environment, providing a concrete means of slowing the advancement of CKD and preventing the impending threat of renal failure. Making wise dietary decisions is a must for controlling renal disease as what we eat can either benefit or damage our kidneys.

Let me introduce you to the **"Stage 3 Kidney Disease Diet Cookbook for Seniors,"** an extensive manual that has been painstakingly created to provide elderly ones with nutrient-dense, doable solutions to help them navigate the intricacies of kidney disease. Inside this book you will find a wealth of tasty, simple-to-follow recipes in these pages that are particularly designed to fulfill the nutritional requirements of seniors living with Stage 3 CKD.

More than a source of food, this book is a reliable ally on the path to improved kidney function and general health. Be prepared to engage in thought-provoking conversations that will clarify the subtleties of chronic kidney disease (CKD), solve the riddles around a renal-friendly diet, and reveal creative methods for grocery shopping and meal planning.

However, this book offers a blueprint for taking back control of one's health destiny rather than merely a compilation of recipes. You will have the information, resources, and motivation necessary to set out on a transforming culinary journey that promises to nurture the body and the spirit with every page you turn. Before you continue to explore the benefits of this book, let me share with you the experience of my two patients whose renal health have been positively transformed via dietary changes and meal plan I presented to them.

"Alice At the age of 75 was dealing with the aftereffects of Stage 3 CKD, which included repeated hospital stays and prescription changes. Resolved to take charge of her health, Alice overhauled her diet, reducing processed and high-potassium meals and concentrating on fresh, natural foods in close collaboration with a nutritionist, Cynthia P. Allison. Alice saw a significant improvement in her kidney function, a decrease in symptoms like weariness and nausea, and a reduction in the need for medication by following her eating plan consistently."

"In addition to being diagnosed with Stage 3 CKD, Robert, who is 70 years old, has been fighting diabetes and high blood pressure. Robert put into practice a thorough diet plan that prioritized portion control, a balance of macronutrients, and mindful eating practices under the direction of his Nutritionist, Cynthia P. Allison. Robert's blood pressure, blood sugar, and renal function all significantly improved with his regular adherence to following his dietary suggestions provided by Cynthia P Allison."

Always have an open mind and an inquisitive mindset while you tackle each dish on your culinary journey. Making careful dietary choices and portion amounts is encouraged, as is experimenting. This cookbook has the potential to be a driving force for good, inspiring you to feel more alive and empowered.

"I am taking proactive steps to manage my kidney health and improve my overall well-being".

1

UNDERSTANDING YOUR KIDNEY

Kidney Function And Filtration

Urine is produced by the kidneys, which are essential for maintaining general health because they filter waste materials and extra fluid from the circulation. The tiny kidney structures known as nephrons are where this filtering process takes place. There are hundreds of nephrons in each kidney, and each one is made up of tubules and glomeruli.

The process of filtering starts in the glomerulus, where blood enters microscopic capillaries with porous walls that hold onto bigger molecules like blood cells and proteins while allowing small molecules like water, electrolytes, and waste items to flow through. The filtrate—a fluid that has been filtered—then passes into the tubules, where waste materials are retained in the tubules to be expelled as urine while vital nutrients and electrolytes are reabsorbed into the circulation.

Maintaining enough hydration, electrolyte balance, and general metabolic function depends on this complex process, which maintains the equilibrium of electrolytes, fluids, and waste products in the body. Any impairment in kidney function may worsen filtration, which can cause the body to retain fluids and poisons and eventually jeopardize health.

How Kidney Mal-function Starts, the Progression of Kidney Disease

A progressive loss of kidney function over time is the hallmark of the complex process of renal disease development. Kidney disease may start off very quietly, with few obvious signs to alert us to the harm that is really taking place within the complex web of renal organs. But when the illness worsens, its effects become more noticeable and there are serious concerns about both immediate health and long-term results.

People may first develop kidney disease in Stages 1 or 2, in which case the renal function is mostly preserved even if there are mild indications of malfunction. However, when the illness advances to Stage 3, there is a more noticeable loss in renal function, which often shows up as higher waste product levels and lower filtration rates. This stage marks a turning point in the development of renal disease and calls for more caution and preventative measures.

If kidney illness in Stage 3 is not treated, it may progress to more severe stages like Stage 4 or Stage 5, when there is a serious danger of renal failure and significantly reduced kidney function. Anemia, electrolyte imbalances, fluid retention, and cardiovascular disease are a few complications that might arise and increase the difficulty of treating the illness.

In the end, kidney disease progression emphasizes how critical it is to identify kidney illness early, monitor it closely, and implement comprehensive treatment strategies that preserve renal function and improve overall health outcomes.

2

INTRODUCTION TO STAGE 3 KIDNEY DISEASE

What is stage 3 CKD (Chronic kidney disease)

A glomerular filtration rate (GFR) of 30 to 59 milliliters per minute per 1.73 square meters is a typical indicator of a significant loss in kidney function in Stage 3 Chronic Kidney Disease (CKD). At this point, people may have a range of symptoms, including dark urine, frequent urination, fluid retention, weakness, exhaustion, sleeplessness, lower back pain, and elevated blood pressure. Still, some people may not exhibit any symptoms. Stage 3a (GFR of 45–59 mL/min) and Stage 3b (GFR of 30–44 mL/min) are the two substages of Stage 3 CKD. The kidneys may continue to carry out their essential tasks despite the impairment in renal function. To stop problems and future deterioration in kidney function, management of Stage 3 CKD focuses on treating underlying risk factors, changing lifestyle, and constantly monitoring kidney function.

Causes and risk factors of stage 3 CKD

The medical illnesses and lifestyle variables that contribute to Stage 3 Chronic Kidney Disease (CKD) are many. Diabetes mellitus, glomerulonephritis, and hypertension are common causes. Aging, smoking, obesity, and a family history of renal disease are possible additional risk factors. Kidney disease may also result from exposure to poisons or pollutants, as well as by taking certain drugs.

Implications of Stage 3 CKD on seniors

Seniors with Chronic Kidney Disease (CKD) in stage 3 have substantial consequences that affect many facets of their health and quality of life. A variety of symptoms, including tiredness, fluid retention, electrolyte imbalances, and anemia, may worsen everyday functioning and quality of life in seniors with Stage 3 CKD as kidney function deteriorates. Furthermore, Stage 3 CKD exacerbates the burden on senior health by raising the risk of comorbidities such as high blood pressure, cardiovascular disease, bone problems, and fluid overload.

Seniors must change their lifestyle and face logistical obstacles while managing Stage 3 CKD, which often calls for food restrictions, drug regimes, and routine medical monitoring. Furthermore, if CKD advances to more severe stages, such as renal failure, intrusive therapies like dialysis or kidney transplantation may be necessary. These procedures may be emotionally and physically exhausting for elderly patients.

Seniors with Stage 3 CKD may also be more susceptible to infection and severe sickness because their bodies are less able to effectively eliminate toxins and maintain proper fluid and electrolyte balance due to impaired kidney function. To maximize their well-being and slow the course of renal disease, seniors with Stage 3 CKD have considerable negative effects on their health overall. This highlights the need for early identification, aggressive treatment, and comprehensive care.

Importance of Early Detection & Intervention

When it comes to the treatment of kidney disease, especially in older adults, early identification and intervention are critical. Early detection of kidney illness enables prompt management to stop complications, decrease the disease's course, and maintain renal function. Early identification allows medical professionals to address underlying risk factors and slow the course of kidney disease by implementing tailored treatment measures, such as dietary changes, medication management, and lifestyle adjustments.

Additionally, early management might lessen the likelihood that kidney disease-related consequences such as anemia, cardiovascular disease, and bone problems would manifest. These complications can have a major negative influence on the health and quality of life of seniors. Healthcare professionals may continuously monitor kidney function, modify treatment strategies as necessary, and provide comprehensive care to meet patients' changing requirements if renal disease is detected early.

Early identification and treatment also lessen the chance that severe kidney disease would need invasive procedures like kidney transplantation or dialysis, which can be emotionally and physically exhausting for elderly patients. Seniors may take charge of their kidney health, maximize treatment results, and enhance their general well-being and lifespan by placing a high priority on early identification and intervention.

Medical Diagnosis and Treatment

A comprehensive strategy is used in the diagnosis and treatment of Stage 3 Chronic Kidney Disease (CKD) with the goals of reducing the disease's development, controlling symptoms, and averting consequences. The process of diagnosing kidney disease usually entails measuring the glomerular filtration rate (GFR) in the blood and evaluating proteinuria and other kidney damage indicators in the urine.

Treatment for underlying causes and risk factors, such as diabetes, hypertension, and lifestyle choices including obesity and smoking, is the main emphasis after a diagnosis. The key to controlling Stage 3 CKD is changing one's lifestyle. This includes quitting smoking, exercising often, and altering one's diet to control electrolyte imbalances and fluid consumption. Medication management is also essential for regulating blood pressure, blood sugar, and other comorbidities to lessen the strain on the kidneys.

Renal function diminishes to the point that sophisticated therapies like dialysis or kidney transplants may become essential in some circumstances. Nevertheless, these therapies are often reserved for advanced CKD stages. To maximize treatment results and maintain kidney health in Stage 3 CKD, regular monitoring of kidney function and close coordination with healthcare professionals is crucial.

Needs for dietary modifications in managing stage 3 CKD

Particularly for elderly patients, dietary changes are essential to the management of renal disease. Seniors may reduce the onset of renal disease, avoid complications, and enhance overall health outcomes by strategically modifying their diet. The usual goals of dietary adjustments are to minimize consumption of potassium, sodium, and phosphorus and to keep an eye on fluid intake to maintain adequate levels of hydration.

Cutting down on salt aids in the management of blood pressure and fluid retention, two frequent issues associated with renal illness. Restricting phosphorus consumption helps avoid mineral imbalances and bone diseases while managing potassium intake helps avoid electrolyte imbalances and irregular cardiac rhythms.

Furthermore, depending on their unique demands and kidney disease stage, seniors with the condition may need to monitor and modify their protein intake. Nutrient-dense meals such as fruits, vegetables, whole grains, and lean meats may be included to improve general health and provide important vitamins and minerals.

Thus, dietary adjustments made to meet the unique requirements of elderly patients with renal disease may have a big influence on how quickly the illness progresses and how well they live. Through close collaboration with healthcare practitioners and certified dietitians, elderly citizens may create customized dietary programs that enhance kidney function and advance their general well-being.

"I honor my body by nourishing it with wholesome foods that support my kidney function and vitality".

3

DIETARY GUIDELINES FOR SENIORS ON STAGE 3 KIDNEY DISEASE

Balancing electrolytes

To prevent complications and slow the development of renal failure, electrolyte balance is essential for the therapy of Stage 3 Chronic Kidney Disease (CKD). Four major electrolyte abnormalities that are often seen in Stage 3 chronic kidney disease (CKD) include **hyperglycemia** (high blood sugar), **hypernatremia** (high salt), **hyperphosphatemia** (high phosphorus), and **hyperkalemia** (high potassium).

Particularly in those with diabetes mellitus, **hyperglycemia** often coexists with chronic kidney disease (CKD) and has to be carefully managed to avoid additional kidney damage and consequences. Regular monitoring, medication management, and dietary changes are among the methods for regulating blood sugar levels.

Hypernatremia may result in fluid retention, elevated blood pressure, and cardiovascular problems since it is caused by poor renal excretion of salt. The three main strategies for treating hypernatremia in Stage 3 CKD are sodium restriction, hydration control, and medication modifications.

Decreased kidney function leads to **hyperphosphatemia**, which is characterized by poor phosphorus excretion. Increased phosphorus levels have been linked to cardiovascular problems, soft tissue calcifications, and bone disease. The management of hyperphosphatemia requires phosphate binders, dietary phosphorus limitation, and careful monitoring of phosphorus levels.

Because decreased kidney function lowers potassium excretion, **hyperkalemia** offers serious hazards for those with chronic renal disease. Elevated potassium levels have the potential to cause arrhythmias in the heart. For the treatment of hyperkalemia in Stage 3 CKD, dietary potassium restriction, medication modifications, and routine potassium level monitoring are essential.

To maximize kidney function and lower the risk of problems, treating electrolyte abnormalities in Stage 3 CKD necessitates a comprehensive strategy that includes dietary adjustments, medication management, and close coordination with healthcare specialists.

Balancing macronutrients

Macronutrient balance is crucial for preserving optimum health and promoting general well-being. Carbohydrates, proteins, and fats are macronutrients that provide the body with energy and are essential for many physiological processes.

The body uses **carbohydrates** as its main energy source to power vital processes like muscular contractions and cognitive activities. Seniors should limit their intake of refined carbohydrates and simple sugars in favor of complex carbs, which include fiber, vitamins, and minerals, such as whole grains, fruits, and vegetables.

Proteins are essential for immune system function, tissue healing, and muscle maintenance. Lean protein sources including fish, chicken, beans, and lentils should be a part of a senior's diet, but consumption should be moderated to prevent undue renal strain.

The synthesis of hormones, the integrity of cell membranes, and the absorption of nutrients all depend on **fats**. Seniors should minimize saturated and trans fats, which are included in processed and fried meals, and emphasize consuming good fats instead, such as those found in avocados, nuts, seeds, and olive oil.

A balanced consumption of macronutrients requires taking each person's dietary requirements, preferences, and health objectives into account. Seniors who want to sustain energy levels, improve metabolism, and encourage satiety should strive to divide macronutrients equally throughout meals and snacks. Seniors may create customized meal plans that satisfy their unique nutritional needs and promote overall health and well-being by speaking with a licensed dietitian.

Balancing Fluid Intake

For numerous body processes to be supported and to be properly hydrated, fluid control is crucial. Elderly people should monitor their fluid intake carefully, particularly if they have Stage 3 Chronic Kidney Disease (CKD), since this may help avoid problems including electrolyte imbalances and fluid overload. Sufficient water promotes healthy renal function, controls body temperature, lubricates joints, and speeds up the transfer of nutrients.

Because reduced kidney function may make it harder to regulate fluid balance, seniors with Stage 3 CKD may need to pay more attention to how much fluid they consume. Limiting fluid consumption in between meals, keeping an eye on the color and flow of urine, and steering clear of salty foods—which may exacerbate fluid retention—are among strategies for managing fluid balance. Nonetheless, it's crucial to collaborate with a medical professional or registered dietitian to create a customized fluid management strategy based on unique requirements and health conditions.

Protein requirements

For seniors, protein is an essential nutrition that supports tissue repair, immunological response, and muscle preservation. To lessen the burden on the kidneys, people with Stage 3 Chronic Kidney Disease (CKD) may need to decrease their protein consumption. Seniors should make an effort to eat a diet rich in lean protein sources, such as fish, chicken, beans, lentils, tofu, and low-fat dairy products.

Seniors with Stage 3 CKD should consume different amounts of protein based on their age, gender, weight, and degree of exercise. The typical daily need for protein is between 0.8 and 1.0 grams per kilogram of body weight. To reduce the risk of future renal damage, seniors with CKD may benefit from a slightly decreased protein consumption.

For general health and well-being, it is crucial to balance the consumption of protein with other macronutrients like **fats and carbs**. Seniors should create a customized meal plan that satisfies their nutritional needs and promotes renal health in collaboration with a certified dietitian or other healthcare professional to ascertain their specific protein requirements. For seniors with Stage 3 CKD, regular renal function monitoring and dietary modifications may be required to maximize health outcomes.

Vitamins and minerals crucial for seniors on stage 3 ckd

Seniors with Stage 3 Chronic Kidney Disease (CKD) have special dietary demands, especially when it comes to vitamins and minerals that are necessary for maintaining general health and controlling the course of the kidney disease. Several important vitamins and minerals are essential for maintaining kidney function and reducing problems related to Stage 3 CKD.

1. Vitamin D: Vitamin D insufficiency is often the result of poor vitamin D metabolism in seniors with Stage 3 CKD. Sufficient amounts of vitamin D are essential for maintaining the immune system, cardiovascular, and bone health. To keep vitamin D levels at their ideal levels, supplements or prescription vitamin D analogs could be required.

2. Calcium: Both muscle and bone health depend on calcium. A calcium imbalance may be more likely in seniors with Stage 3 CKD because of their compromised renal function. To avoid consequences like bone disease and cardiovascular problems, it may be important to monitor calcium levels and regulate consumption by dietary adjustments or supplementation.

3. Iron: Because CKD reduces the synthesis of erythropoietin, a hormone that is necessary for the development of red blood cells, iron deficiency anemia is often seen. Seniors with Stage 3 CKD need to make sure they are getting enough iron from foods like beans, fish, poultry, lean meats, and fortified cereals. In circumstances when the deficit is severe, iron supplements may be recommended.

4. B vitamins: B vitamins, which include folate, B12, and B6, are crucial for red blood cell formation, energy metabolism, and neuron function. B vitamin absorption may be compromised in seniors with Stage 3 CKD as a result of gastrointestinal problems or drug interactions. B vitamin deficits may be avoided and general health can be supported by routinely checking B vitamin levels and supplementing as necessary.

5. Potassium and phosphorus: To avoid electrolyte imbalances and consequences like hyperkalemia and hyperphosphatemia, seniors with Stage 3 CKD should keep an eye on their intake of potassium and phosphorus. It may be essential to adjust medication and diet to keep potassium and phosphorus levels within the advised range.

To sustain kidney function, avoid problems, and enhance general well-being, seniors with Stage 3 CKD must maintain appropriate vitamin and mineral status. Developing individualized food programs and supplement schedules that are suited to each person's requirements and health condition requires close observation of nutritional status and close coordination with healthcare experts.

Daily Nutrient Recommendation for Seniors on Stage 3 CKD

Nutrient	Recommended Daily Limit
Sodium	Less than 2,000 mg per day
Phosphorus	Less than 800-1,000 mg per day (varies based on individual needs)
Potassium	Varies based on individual needs; typically 2,000-3,000 mg per day
Protein	0.8-1.0 grams per kilogram of body weight per day
Fluids	Limit based on individual needs and urine output
Vitamin D	Consult healthcare provider for supplementation recommendations
Calcium	800-1,200 mg per day (considering individual calcium and phosphate levels)
Iron	8-18 mg per day (varies based on gender and individual needs)
B Vitamins (B12, B6, Folate)	Meet recommended dietary allowances (RDAs)

Positive Affirmations for Seniors with Stage 3 Kidney Disease

"I am worthy of love, care, and attention, including prioritizing my dietary and lifestyle needs".

4

ESSENTIAL KITCHEN PRACTICES FOR SENIORS ON STAGE 3 CKD

Basic Required Kitchen Tools

Having specific kitchen appliances and equipment that make meal preparation easier and meet nutritional requirements might be beneficial for seniors with Stage 3 Chronic Kidney Disease (CKD). For seniors with Stage 3 CKD, the following are necessary kitchen tools:

1. Food Scale: When measuring portion sizes, particularly for items like meats, fruits, and vegetables that may need close attention to their protein, potassium, and phosphorus levels, a food scale may be very helpful to seniors.

2. Measuring Cups and Spoons: When following recipes or dietary recommendations, portion management and precise ingredient measurement depend on measuring cups and spoons.

3. Blender or Food Processor: Seniors with CKD might find it easier to eat nutrient-rich meals like fruits and vegetables by using a blender or food processor to make healthy smoothies, purees, and soups.

4. Nonstick cookware: Nonstick Cookware lowers the need for additional fats and oils while cooking, which makes it simpler to follow dietary guidelines for controlling fat consumption.

5. Vegetable Steamer: Using a vegetable steamer, seniors may cook veggies while maintaining their natural taste and nutritional worth without using too much salt or oil.

6. The Instant Pot and Slow Cooker are two multipurpose kitchen tools that seniors may use to prepare meals easily and save time and energy by cooking a range of foods with little effort.

Ingredients and Pantry Staples

Seniors with Stage 3 Chronic Kidney Disease (CKD) should make it a priority to buy items that meet their nutritional requirements and dietary restrictions to begin preparing kidney-friendly meals. Important components consist of:

1. Lean Proteins: Opt for lean protein sources including lentils, beans, skinless chicken, fish, and tofu. These choices are appropriate for CKD diets since they are low in potassium and phosphorus.

2. Whole Grains: Choose whole grains that are high in fiber and critical nutrients without being too salted or phosphorus-rich, such as brown rice, quinoa, barley, and whole wheat pasta.

3. Fresh Fruits and Vegetables: Choose a range of fresh fruits and vegetables, with an emphasis on low-potassium varieties such as green beans, apples, berries, cabbage, and cauliflower. These selections are kidney-friendly and high in vitamins, minerals, and antioxidants.

4. Low-Sodium Condiments and Seasonings: Instead of using high-sodium condiments to flavor food, try using herbs, spices, vinegar, and lemon juice. Select sauces such as tomato sauce, salad dressings, and soy sauce that are reduced in sodium or contain no salt.

5. Dairy Alternatives: Use low-phosphorus substitutes in place of dairy products, such as rice milk, almond milk, and nondairy yogurt. These choices provide you with protein and calcium without adding to your phosphorus excess.

Ingredients Substitution

For seniors with Stage 3 Chronic Kidney Disease (CKD), it is essential to make necessary ingredient replacements so they may still enjoy tasty and nourishing meals while adhering to their dietary limitations. The following are some typical ingredient swaps for CKD-friendly cooking:

1. Salt Substitutes: To add taste to food without adding more sodium to the diet, use herbs, spices, and mixes of seasonings instead of table salt.

2. Low-Potassium veggies: To control potassium levels, swap out high-potassium veggies like potatoes, tomatoes, and spinach for lower-potassium ones like bell peppers, cucumbers, and cauliflower.

3. Phosphorus-Free Dairy Alternatives: To avoid phosphorus accumulation in the blood, substitute phosphorus-free dairy products such as almond milk, rice milk, and non-dairy cheese with dairy items with a high phosphorus concentration, including milk and cheese.

4. Whole Grain Substitutes: To boost fiber consumption and promote general health without going above phosphorus restrictions, use whole grain substitutes like brown rice, quinoa, and whole wheat pasta in place of refined grains.

5. Lean Protein Sources: To minimize phosphorus and saturated fat consumption while still achieving protein requirements, choose lean protein sources such as skinless chicken, fish, tofu, and lentils rather than high-fat meats.

Seniors with Stage 3 CKD may enjoy tasty, kidney-friendly meals that meet their nutritional needs and support optimum renal function by substituting these ingredients. A certified dietitian or other healthcare professional should always be consulted for individualized advice on ingredient replacements based on specific nutritional requirements and preferences.

Cooking Techniques Suitable for Seniors with Stage 3 Kidney Disease

Seniors with Stage 3 Chronic Kidney Disease (CKD) should cook with an emphasis on convenience, simplicity, and safety, but without sacrificing taste and nutrition. Seniors may benefit from the following culinary techniques:

1. Steaming: Steaming is a low-fat, low-sodium cooking technique that maintains food's natural tastes and minerals. With a steamer basket or microwave steamer, seniors may quickly steam fish, chicken, and vegetables with little assistance or supervision.

2. Boiling: Boiling is a simple cooking method in which foods are cooked thoroughly by immersing them in boiling water. This approach may be used by seniors to ensure that vegetables and legumes are soft and simple to digest, as well as grains like pasta and rice.

3. Baking: Baking is a hands-off cooking method that uses dry heat to cook food in an oven. Seniors may bake a wide range of foods by just putting them in a prepared oven and cooking them until they are soft and golden brown. Examples of baked foods include casseroles, baked fish or poultry, and roasted vegetables.

4. Slow Cooking: Slow cooking is a practical cooking technique that entails letting items stew for a long time on low heat in a crockpot or slow cooker. This approach requires less preparation and supervision for seniors to make robust soups, stews, and tender meats.

5. Microwave: Seniors may quickly and effectively make meals in the microwave in a matter of minutes. The microwave is a great tool for seniors with limited movement or energy since it can be used to bake potatoes, steam vegetables, cook cereals, and reheat leftovers.

Seniors with Stage 3 CKD may effortlessly produce wholesome meals that fulfill their cravings and meet their nutritional requirements by using these culinary skills. Additionally, seniors may keep their freedom and enjoy home-cooked meals with little effort by using kitchen appliances like microwaves and slow cookers, as well as combining pre-prepared items.

Tips on Reducing Nutrients on Every Day Meals

Seniors with Stage 3 Chronic Kidney Disease (CKD) may lower the amount of specific nutrients, such as potassium, phosphorus, and sodium, in their regular meals by using useful tactics and advice that encourage kidney-friendly dietary habits:

1. *study Labels:* Seniors should carefully study food labels to detect substances that are rich in potassium, phosphorus, and salt. When feasible, they should pick lower-sodium or phosphorus-free alternatives.

2. *Select Fresh Foods:* Avoid processed or packaged foods, which often have high salt, phosphorus, and potassium levels, and instead choose fresh fruits, vegetables, and lean meats. Fresh foods include vital vitamins, minerals, and antioxidants and are naturally lower in these nutrients.

3. *Rinse Canned Foods:* To lower the salt level, rinse canned fruits, vegetables, and beans under cold water before eating. By taking this easy step, the extra salt from the canning process may be eliminated, improving the renal friendliness of the food.

4. *Use Herbs and Spices:* To improve flavor without adding more sodium to your diet, add herbs, spices, vinegar, lemon juice, and other low-sodium seasonings to your food in place of salt. Trying out new taste combinations may add a lot of enjoyment and satisfaction to meals.

5. Reduce Your Consumption of Processed Meats: Because these meats are rich in salt, phosphorus, and potassium, try to cut down on your intake of hot dogs, bacon, sausage, and deli meats. Instead, go for plant-based protein substitutes like tofu and lentils or fresh, unprocessed meats.

6. Use Portion Control: Keep an eye on serving sizes to prevent overindulging and lower consumption of nutrients like potassium and phosphorus. Controlling portion sizes and preventing excessive nutrient intake may be achieved by using smaller plates, quantifying quantities using measuring cups or a food scale and refraining from second helpings.

Seniors with Stage 3 CKD may successfully lower their daily meal consumption of salt, phosphorus, and potassium by implementing these useful guidelines, which will improve renal health and general well-being.

Meal Planning and Portion Management

For seniors with Stage 3 Chronic Kidney Disease (CKD), portion management and meal planning are crucial elements of a kidney-friendly diet that will help them regulate their nutritional intake, reduce their symptoms, and maintain overall kidney function. Seniors may make meal planning and portion management a regular habit by following these tips:

1. Portion Control:

Use Smaller dishes: To manage portion sizes and avoid overindulging, use smaller dishes and bowls. Seniors may find that lesser portions satisfy them more when they use this visual cue.

Measure: To ensure that portions of high-protein foods like meat and dairy, which should be taken in moderation, are precisely measured, use measuring cups, spoons, and a food scale.

To avoid overeating and encourage improved digestion, practice mindful eating by taking your time at meals, chewing your food fully, and paying attention to your body's signals of hunger and fullness.

Split Meals: To manage portion sizes and save calories while eating out, think about dividing entrée with a companion or bringing half of the meal home for later.

2. Organizing Meals:

Make a Plan: Allocate a certain period every week to strategize meals and snacks, considering dietary limitations, nutritional requirements, and individual choices. Make a shopping list based on your meal plans to make sure you have everything you need.

Select Foods That Are Good for Your Kidneys: Make an effort to include foods that are good for your kidneys in your meals and snacks, such as fruits, vegetables, lean meats, and whole grains. Eat less or stay away from foods heavy in potassium, phosphorus, and salt.

Plan Ahead: To save time and guarantee you have healthy alternatives on hand, cook in bulk and prepare meals ahead of time. For convenient grab-and-go choices, portion meals into individual portions and keep them in the freezer or refrigerator.

Seek Variety: To make sure you're receiving a broad range of nutrients, include a variety of foods from various food categories in your meals and snacks. To keep meals engaging and fun, try out different tastes and dishes.

Label-reading Techniques

For seniors with Stage 3 Chronic Kidney Disease (CKD), reading food labels is essential to making educated dietary decisions. Among the methods for interpreting labels are:

1. Examine Serving Size: The number of nutrients per serving is determined by the serving size specified on the nutrition label. To be sure you are getting the right amount of nutrients, compare the serving size to the quantity you usually eat.

2. Examine the Nutrient Content: Find out about potassium, salt, phosphorus, and other nutrients that are important for kidney health. Select goods that are lower in these nutrients.

3. Scan Ingredients List: Look for high-sodium additions such as sodium nitrate, monosodium glutamate (MSG), and salt in the ingredients list. Steer clear of goods that include phosphorus additions, such as phosphoric acid and phosphate.

4. Select Whole Foods: Go for whole, unprocessed foods that have less added sugar, salt, and potassium and fewer additional components overall.

5. Marketing promises to Be Wary of: Be wary of promises made in the marketing that something is "low-fat" or "reduced-sodium," since these products may still contain substantial levels of other dangerous components.

6. Compare items: Look for the product that has the least amount of sodium, phosphorus, potassium, and other potentially harmful nutrients by comparing comparable items. To promote kidney health, wherever feasible, choose items with a reduced nutritional content.

7. Use Smartphone applications: To get nutritional data and ingredient lists for a variety of food items, think about using internet databases or smartphone applications. Seniors using these materials may plan their meals and shop with more knowledge.

5

KIDNEY-FRIENDLY RECIPES FOR SENIORS ON STAGE 3 KIDNEY DISEASE

BREAKFAST

Veggie Omelette

Preparation Time: 10 minutes
Cooking Time: 10 minutes
Servings: 2

Ingredients:
- 4 eggs
- 1/4 cup diced bell peppers
- 1/4 cup diced onions
- 1/4 cup chopped spinach
- 1/4 cup shredded low-fat cheese
- Salt and pepper to taste

Instructions:
1. Beat the eggs in a bowl until well combined.
2. Add the chopped onions, bell peppers, and spinach to a nonstick pan set over medium heat. Sauté the veggies until they are soft.

3. Evenly cover the veggies in the skillet with the beaten eggs.
4. After the omelette has been cooked until the eggs are set, sprinkle the shredded cheese on top.
5. Fold the omelette in half and serve hot.

Nutritional Values (per serving):

Calories: 180
Protein: 14g
Carbohydrates: 5g
Fat: 12g
Potassium: 320mg
Sodium: 320mg
Phosphorus: 180mg

Overnight Oats

Preparation Time: 5 minutes
Cooking Time: 0 minutes
Servings: 2

Ingredients:
- 1 cup rolled oats
- 1 cup unsweetened almond milk
- 1/2 cup Greek yogurt
- 1 tablespoon chia seeds
- 1 cup mixed berries
- 1 tablespoon honey or maple syrup (optional)

Instructions:
1. Place rolled oats, Greek yogurt, almond milk, and chia seeds in a dish or container. Mix well by stirring.

2. Store the jar or dish in the refrigerator for the whole night.
3. Add mixed berries to the oats in the morning and, if you'd like, sprinkle with honey or maple syrup.
4. Stir before serving.

Nutritional Values (per serving):

Calories: 250
Protein: 12g
Carbohydrates: 35g
Fat: 7g
Potassium: 250mg
Sodium: 100mg
Phosphorus: 180mg

Greek Yogurt Parfait

Preparation Time: 5 minutes
Cooking Time: 0 minutes
Servings: 1

Ingredients:
- 1/2 cup Greek yogurt
- 1/4 cup mixed berries
- 1 tablespoon chopped almonds or walnuts
- 1 teaspoon honey or maple syrup (optional)

Instructions:
1. Arrange Greek yogurt, chopped almonds, and mixed berries in a glass or dish.
2. If preferred, drizzle with maple syrup or honey.
3. Serve immediately.

Nutritional Values (per serving):

Calories: 180
Protein: 15g
Carbohydrates: 20g
Fat: 6g
Potassium: 220mg
Sodium: 80mg
Phosphorus: 180mg

Avocado Toast

Preparation Time: 5 minutes
Cooking Time: 0 minutes
Servings: 1

Ingredients:

- 1 slice whole grain bread
- 1/2 avocado, mashed
- Salt and pepper to taste
- Optional toppings: sliced tomatoes, red pepper flakes, sliced hard-boiled egg

Instructions:

1. Toast the whole grain bread slice until it becomes golden brown.
2. Evenly distribute the mashed avocado on the bread.
3. To taste, add salt and pepper for seasoning.
4. Top with optional toppings if desired.
5. Serve immediately.

Nutritional Values (per serving):

Calories: 200	Protein: 5g	Carbohydrates: 15g
Fat: 15g	Potassium: 380mg	
Sodium: 150mg	Phosphorus: 150mg	

Breakfast Burrito

Preparation Time: 10 minutes
Cooking Time: 10 minutes
Servings: 2

Ingredients:
- 2 large whole wheat tortillas
- 4 eggs, beaten
- 1/4 cup black beans, drained and rinsed
- 1/4 cup diced tomatoes
- 1/4 cup diced bell peppers
- 1/4 cup shredded low-fat cheese
- Salt and pepper to taste
- Optional toppings: salsa, avocado slices, Greek yogurt

Instructions:
1. Scramble the beaten eggs in a pan until they are fully done.
2. Use a skillet or microwave to reheat the whole wheat tortillas.
3. Evenly distribute the shredded cheese, diced tomatoes, diced bell peppers, black beans, scrambled eggs, and black beans among the tortillas.
4. To taste, add salt and pepper for seasoning.
5. Create burritos by rolling up the tortillas.
6. Serve with optional toppings if desired.

Nutritional Values (per serving):

Calories: 300

Protein: 20g

Carbohydrates: 25g

Fat: 12g

Potassium: 350mg

Sodium: 400mg   Phosphorus: 200mg

Quinoa Breakfast Bowl

Preparation Time: 15 minutes
Cooking Time: 15 minutes
Servings: 2

Ingredients:

- 1/2 cup quinoa, rinsed
- 1 cup water or low-sodium vegetable broth
- 1/2 cup diced mango or pineapple
- 1/4 cup sliced almonds
- 1 tablespoon honey or maple syrup (optional)

Instructions:

1. Bring water or vegetable broth to a boil in a saucepan.
2. Turn down the heat to low and add the rinsed quinoa. Once the quinoa is cooked and the water has been absorbed, cover and simmer for 15 minutes.
3. Use a fork to fluff the quinoa and distribute it into serving dishes.
4. Add sliced almonds and chopped mango or pineapple on top.
5. If preferred, drizzle with maple syrup or honey.
6. Serve warm.

Nutritional Values (per serving):

Calories: 300

Protein: 10g

Carbohydrates: 50g

Fat: 8g

Potassium: 250mg

Sodium: 10mg

Phosphorus: 180mg

Spinach and Feta Frittata Muffins

Preparation Time: 10 minutes
Cooking Time: 20 minutes
Servings: 4

Ingredients:
- 6 eggs
- 1 cup chopped spinach
- 1/4 cup crumbled feta cheese
- Salt and pepper to taste

Instructions:
1. Oil a muffin tray and preheat the oven to 350°F (175°C).
2. Beat the eggs well in a basin.
3. Add the crumbled feta cheese and chopped spinach. Add pepper and salt for seasoning.
4. Fill each cup of the muffin tray approximately 3/4 of the way to the top with the egg mixture.
5. Bake the frittata muffins for 20 minutes, or until they are gently brown and firm.
6. Allow to cool slightly before serving.

Nutritional Values (per serving):
Calories: 150

Protein: 10g

Carbohydrates: 2g

Fat: 10g

Potassium: 200mg

Sodium: 180mg

Phosphorus: 150mg

Berry Smoothie

Preparation Time: 5 minutes
Cooking Time: 0 minutes
Servings: 1

Ingredients:

- 1/2 cup mixed berries (such as strawberries, blueberries, raspberries)
- 1/2 cup spinach leaves
- 1/2 cup unsweetened almond milk
- 1/4 cup Greek yogurt
- 1 tablespoon chia seeds
- 1 teaspoon honey or maple syrup (optional)

Instructions:

1. Put mixed berries, spinach leaves, Greek yogurt, almond milk, and chia seeds in a blender.
2. Blend until creamy and smooth.
3. If desired, add honey or maple syrup to taste and sweeten.
4. Present right away.

Nutritional Values (per serving):

Calories: 150

Protein: 8g

Carbohydrates: 20g

Fat: 5g

Potassium: 250mg

Sodium: 100mg

Phosphorus: 180mg

Cottage Cheese Pancakes

Preparation Time: 10 minutes
Cooking Time: 10 minutes
Servings: 2

Ingredients:

- 1 cup cottage cheese
- 2 eggs
- 1/4 cup almond flour or oat flour
- 1 teaspoon vanilla extract
- 1/2 teaspoon cinnamon
- Optional toppings: sliced bananas, berries, Greek yogurt

Instructions:

1. Put almond flour, eggs, cinnamon, vanilla extract, and cottage cheese in a blender. Process till smooth.
2. Apply a thin layer of cooking spray and preheat a nonstick skillet over medium heat.
3. To make little pancakes, pour the pancake batter into the griddle.
4. Cook until cooked through and golden brown, 2 to 3 minutes each side.
5. If preferred, garnish hot dish with optional toppings.

Nutritional Values (per serving):

Calories: 250

Protein: 25g

Carbohydrates: 10g

Fat: 10g

Potassium: 300mg

Sodium: 400mg

Phosphorus: 250mg

Breakfast Bowl with Sweet Potatoes

Preparation Time: 15 minutes
Cooking Time: 25 minutes
Servings: 2

Ingredients:

- 1 large sweet potato, diced
- 1 tablespoon olive oil
- 1/2 teaspoon paprika
- Salt and pepper to taste
- 4 eggs
- 1/4 cup shredded cheese
- Optional toppings: diced avocado, salsa, Greek yogurt

Instructions:

1. Line a baking sheet with parchment paper and preheat the oven to 400°F (200°C).
2. Combine the sweet potatoes, diced, olive oil, paprika, salt, and pepper in a basin.
3. Arrange the sweet potatoes on the prepared baking sheet in a single layer, and roast for 20 to 25 minutes, or until they are soft and have a golden brown color.
4. In the meanwhile, prepare the eggs as desired (scrambled, fried, poached).
5. Spoon the roasted sweet potatoes into serving dishes, then top with shredded cheese and fried eggs.
6. If preferred, garnish hot dish with optional toppings.

Nutritional Values (per serving):

Calories: 300

Protein: 15g

Carbohydrates: 25g

Fat: 15g

Potassium: 450mg

Sodium: 200mg

Phosphorus: 200mg

Positive Affirmations for Seniors with Stage 3 Kidney Disease

"I choose to focus on what I can control and let go of worry about things beyond my control".

LUNCH

Grilled Chicken Salad

Preparation Time: 15 minutes
Cooking Time: 15 minutes
Servings: 4

Ingredients:

- 1 lb boneless, skinless chicken breasts
- 8 cups mixed salad greens
- 1 cup cherry tomatoes, halved
- 1 cucumber, sliced
- 1/2 red onion, thinly sliced
- 1/4 cup sliced almonds
- 1/4 cup balsamic vinaigrette

Instructions:

1. Preheat grill to medium-high heat.
2. Season chicken breasts with salt and pepper, then grill for 6-7 minutes per side until cooked through.
3. Let chicken rest for 5 minutes, then slice.
4. In a large bowl, toss together salad greens, cherry tomatoes, cucumber, red onion, and sliced almonds.
5. Divide salad among plates, top with sliced grilled chicken, and drizzle with balsamic vinaigrette.

Nutritional Values (per serving):

Calories: 300   Protein: 25g
Carbohydrates: 15g   Fat: 15g
Potassium: 400mg   Sodium: 250mg   Phosphorus: 200mg

Lentil Soup

Preparation Time: 10 minutes
Cooking Time: 45 minutes
Servings: 6

Ingredients:

- 1 cup dried lentils, rinsed
- 1 onion, diced
- 2 carrots, diced
- 2 celery stalks, diced
- 4 cups vegetable broth
- 1 can (14 oz) diced tomatoes
- 2 cloves garlic, minced
- 1 teaspoon dried thyme
- Salt and pepper to taste

Instructions:

1. In a large pot, sauté onion, carrots, and celery until softened.
2. Add minced garlic and cook for 1 minute.
3. Stir in dried lentils, vegetable broth, diced tomatoes, and dried thyme.
4. Bring to a boil, then reduce heat and simmer for 30-40 minutes until lentils are tender.
5. Season with salt and pepper to taste before serving.

Nutritional Values (per serving):

Calories: 200

Protein: 12g

Carbohydrates: 30g

Fat: 2g

Potassium: 300mg

Sodium: 400mg   Phosphorus: 180mg

Tuna Salad Wrap

Preparation Time: 10 minutes
Cooking Time: 0 minutes
Servings: 2

Ingredients:

- 1 can (5 oz) tuna, drained
- 1/4 cup Greek yogurt
- 1 tablespoon lemon juice
- 1/4 cup diced celery
- 1/4 cup diced red onion
- 2 whole wheat tortillas
- 1 cup **mixed salad greens**

Instructions:

1. In a bowl, mix together drained tuna, Greek yogurt, lemon juice, diced celery, and diced red onion.
2. Place a tortilla on a flat surface and spread half of the tuna salad mixture onto it.
3. Top with mixed salad greens, then roll up tightly.
4. Repeat with remaining ingredients to make the second wrap.
5. Slice wraps in half and serve.

Nutritional Values (per serving):

Calories: 250

Protein: 20g

Carbohydrates: 25g

Fat: 8g

Potassium: 300mg

Sodium: 350mg

Phosphorus: 200mg

Quinoa Salad with Roasted Vegetables

Preparation Time: 15 minutes
Cooking Time: 25 minutes
Servings: 4

Ingredients:

- 1 cup quinoa, rinsed
- 2 cups mixed vegetables (such as bell peppers, zucchini, eggplant), diced
- 2 tablespoons olive oil
- 1 teaspoon dried herbs (such as thyme, rosemary)
- Salt and pepper to taste
- 1/4 cup feta cheese, crumbled
- 2 tablespoons balsamic vinegar

Instructions:

1. Preheat oven to 400°F (200°C) and line a baking sheet with parchment paper.
2. Toss diced mixed vegetables with olive oil, dried herbs, salt, and pepper on the baking sheet.
3. Roast vegetables for 20-25 minutes until tender and lightly browned.
4. Meanwhile, cook quinoa according to package instructions.
5. In a large bowl, combine cooked quinoa, roasted vegetables, crumbled feta cheese, and balsamic vinegar. Mix well.
6. Serve warm or cold.

Nutritional Values (per serving):

Calories: 280	Protein: 8g
Carbohydrates: 35g	Fat: 12g
Potassium: 350mg	Sodium: 250mg
Phosphorus: 180mg	

Turkey and Veggie Sandwich on Whole Wheat Bread

Preparation Time: 10 minutes
Cooking Time: 0 minutes
Servings: 2

Ingredients:

- 4 slices whole wheat bread
- 4 oz sliced turkey breast
- 1/2 avocado, sliced
- 1/2 cup mixed salad greens
- 1/4 cup sliced cucumber
- 1/4 cup sliced tomato
- 2 tablespoons hummus

Instructions:

1. Toast the slices of whole wheat bread if desired.
2. Spread hummus evenly on each slice of bread.
3. Layer sliced turkey breast, avocado, mixed salad greens, cucumber, and tomato on two slices of bread.
4. Top with the remaining slices of bread to make sandwiches.
5. Slice sandwiches in half and serve.

Nutritional Values (per serving):

Calories: 300

Protein: 20g

Carbohydrates: 25g

Fat: 12g

Potassium: 400mg

Sodium: 350mg

Phosphorus: 200mg

Vegetable Stir-Fry with Brown Rice

Preparation Time: 15 minutes
Cooking Time: 15 minutes
Servings: 4

Ingredients:

- 2 cups cooked brown rice
- 2 tablespoons sesame oil
- 2 cloves garlic, minced
- 1 tablespoon grated ginger
- 1 bell pepper, sliced
- 1 cup broccoli florets
- 1 cup sliced mushrooms
- 1 carrot, julienned
- 1/4 cup low-sodium soy sauce
- 1 tablespoon rice vinegar
- 1 tablespoon honey or maple syrup

Instructions:

1. Heat sesame oil in a large skillet or wok over medium-high heat.
2. Add minced garlic and grated ginger, stir-fry for 30 seconds.
3. Add sliced bell pepper, broccoli florets, sliced mushrooms, and julienned carrot. Stir-fry for 5-7 minutes until vegetables are tender-crisp.
4. In a small bowl, mix together low-sodium soy sauce, rice vinegar, and honey or maple syrup.
5. Pour the sauce over the stir-fried vegetables and toss to coat evenly.
6. Serve the vegetable stir-fry over cooked brown rice.

Nutritional Values (per serving):

Calories: 250   Protein: 8g   Carbohydrates: 40g   Fat: 8g

Potassium: 300mg   Sodium: 400mg   Phosphorus: 180mg

Chickpea Salad with Feta and Cucumber

Preparation Time: 10 minutes
Cooking Time: 0 minutes
Servings: 4

Ingredients:
- 1 can (15 oz) chickpeas, drained and rinsed
- 1 cucumber, diced
- 1/4 cup diced red onion
- 1/4 cup crumbled feta cheese
- 2 tablespoons chopped fresh parsley
- 2 tablespoons olive oil
- 1 tablespoon lemon juice
- Salt and pepper to taste

Instructions:
1. In a large bowl, combine chickpeas, diced cucumber, diced red onion, crumbled feta cheese, and chopped fresh parsley.
2. Drizzle with olive oil and lemon juice, then season with salt and pepper.
3. Toss to coat evenly.
4. Serve chilled or at room temperature.

Nutritional Values (per serving):

Calories: 200

Protein: 8g

Carbohydrates: 20g

Fat: 10g

Potassium: 250mg

Sodium: 300mg

Phosphorus: 180mg

Salmon and Avocado Sushi Bowl

Preparation Time: 20 minutes
Cooking Time: 10 minutes
Servings: 2

Ingredients:

- 1 cup sushi rice, cooked
- 2 salmon fillets, cooked and flaked
- 1 avocado, sliced
- 1/2 cucumber, sliced
- 1/4 cup shredded nori seaweed
- 2 tablespoons low-sodium soy sauce
- 1 tablespoon rice vinegar
- 1 teaspoon sesame oil
- 1 teaspoon sesame seeds

Instructions:

1. Divide cooked sushi rice between serving bowls.
2. Arrange cooked and flaked salmon, sliced avocado, sliced cucumber, and shredded nori seaweed on top of the rice.
3. In a small bowl, mix together low-sodium soy sauce, rice vinegar, sesame oil, and sesame seeds.
4. Drizzle the sauce over the sushi bowls.
5. Serve immediately.

Nutritional Values (per serving):

Calories: 300

Protein: 20g

Carbohydrates: 30g

Fat: 12g   Potassium: 400mg

Sodium: 300mg   Phosphorus: 250mg

Black Bean Quesadilla with Guacamole

Preparation Time: 10 minutes
Cooking Time: 10 minutes
Servings: 2

Ingredients:
- 4 whole wheat tortillas
- 1 can (15 oz) black beans, drained and rinsed
- 1/2 cup shredded cheddar cheese
- 1 avocado, mashed
- 1/4 cup diced tomato
- 1/4 cup diced red onion
- 1 tablespoon lime juice
- 1/4 teaspoon cumin
- Salt and pepper to taste

Instructions:
1. Preheat a non-stick skillet over medium heat.
2. Place one tortilla in the skillet and sprinkle with half of the shredded cheddar cheese.
3. Spoon half of the black beans evenly over the cheese.
4. Top with another tortilla and cook until the bottom tortilla is golden brown and crispy, about 3-4 minutes.
5. Flip the quesadilla and cook the other side until golden brown and crispy, another 3-4 minutes.
6. Meanwhile, in a bowl, mix together mashed avocado, diced tomato, diced red onion, lime juice, cumin, salt, and pepper to make guacamole.
7. Remove quesadilla from the skillet and slice into wedges. Serve with guacamole on the side.

Nutritional Values (per serving):

Calories: 300

Protein: 15g

Carbohydrates: 35g

Fat: 12g

Potassium: 350mg

Sodium: 350mg

Phosphorus: 200mg

Greek Salad with Grilled Shrimp

Preparation Time: 20 minutes
Cooking Time: 10 minutes
Servings: 2

Ingredients:

- 1/2 lb large shrimp, peeled and deveined
- 2 cups mixed salad greens
- 1/2 cucumber, diced
- 1/2 cup cherry tomatoes, halved
- 1/4 cup sliced red onion
- 1/4 cup crumbled feta cheese
- 2 tablespoons kalamata olives, pitted
- 2 tablespoons extra virgin olive oil
- 1 tablespoon red wine vinegar
- 1 teaspoon dried oregano
- Salt and pepper to taste

Instructions:

1. Preheat grill to medium-high heat.
2. Thread shrimp onto skewers and season with salt, pepper, and dried oregano.
3. Grill shrimp for 2-3 minutes per side until pink and cooked through.
4. In a large bowl, toss together mixed salad greens, diced cucumber, halved cherry tomatoes, sliced red onion, crumbled feta cheese, and pitted kalamata olives.
5. In a small bowl, whisk together extra virgin olive oil, red wine vinegar, and a pinch of dried oregano to make the dressing.
6. Drizzle dressing over the salad and toss to coat evenly.
7. Divide salad among plates and top with grilled shrimp.

Nutritional Values (per serving):

Calories: 300
Protein: 20g
Carbohydrates: 15g
Fat: 18g
Potassium: 400mg
Sodium: 350mg
Phosphorus: 250mg

"I am empowered to make informed decisions about my health and advocate for myself in my healthcare journey".

DINNER

Baked Salmon with Lemon and Herbs

Preparation Time: 10 minutes
Cooking Time: 15 minutes
Servings: 4

Ingredients:

- 4 salmon fillets
- 2 tablespoons olive oil
- 2 cloves garlic, minced
- 1 lemon, sliced
- 1 tablespoon fresh dill, chopped
- Salt and pepper to taste

Instructions:

1. Preheat oven to 375°F (190°C) and line a baking sheet with parchment paper.
2. Place salmon fillets on the prepared baking sheet.
3. Drizzle olive oil over the salmon, then sprinkle minced garlic, chopped dill, salt, and pepper on top.
4. Place lemon slices on top of the salmon fillets.
5. Bake in the preheated oven for 12-15 minutes until salmon is cooked through and flakes easily with a fork.

Nutritional Values (per serving):

Calories: 250	Protein: 25g
Carbohydrates: 1g	Fat: 15g
Potassium: 400mg	Sodium: 100mg
Phosphorus: 250mg	

Chicken Stir-Fry with Broccoli and Bell Peppers

Preparation Time: 15 minutes
Cooking Time: 15 minutes
Servings: 4

Ingredients:

- 1 lb boneless, skinless chicken breasts, thinly sliced
- 2 cups broccoli florets
- 1 red bell pepper, sliced
- 1 yellow bell pepper, sliced
- 2 tablespoons soy sauce
- 1 tablespoon hoisin sauce
- 1 tablespoon sesame oil
- 2 cloves garlic, minced
- 1 teaspoon grated ginger

Instructions:

1. In a large skillet or wok, heat the sesame oil over medium-high heat.
2. Stir-fry the grated ginger and minced garlic for 30 seconds.
3. Place the cut chicken breasts in the pan and cook them thoroughly and browned.
4. Add the sliced bell peppers and broccoli florets to the pan and stir-fry for 5 to 7 minutes, or until the veggies are crisp-tender.
5. Stir in soy sauce and hoisin sauce, toss to coat evenly.
6. Serve hot.

Nutritional Values (per serving):

Calories: 300   Protein: 30g
Carbohydrates: 10g   Fat: 15g
Potassium: 450mg   Sodium: 400mg
Phosphorus: 300mg

Vegetable Curry with Tofu

Preparation Time: 20 minutes
Cooking Time: 25 minutes
Servings: 4

Ingredients:

- 1 block (14 oz) firm tofu, cubed
- 2 cups mixed vegetables (such as carrots, peas, bell peppers, cauliflower)
- 1 onion, chopped
- 2 cloves garlic, minced
- 1 can (14 oz) coconut milk
- 2 tablespoons curry powder
- 1 tablespoon olive oil
- Salt and pepper to taste

Instructions:

1. In a big skillet over medium heat, warm up the olive oil.
2. Add the minced garlic and onion and sauté until softened.
3. In the pan, add the cubed tofu and cook until it becomes golden brown on both sides.
4. Cook for five minutes after adding the curry powder and mixed veggies.
5. After adding the coconut milk, boil the veggies for a further ten minutes, or until they are soft.
6. To taste, add salt and pepper for seasoning.
7. Serve warm with naan bread or rice.

Nutritional Values (per serving):

Calories: 280   Protein: 15g   Carbohydrates: 15g
Fat: 20g   Potassium: 350mg
Sodium: 200mg   Phosphorus: 200mg

Turkey Meatballs with Whole Wheat Pasta

Preparation Time: 20 minutes
Cooking Time: 20 minutes
Servings: 4

Ingredients:

- 1 lb lean ground turkey
- 1/4 cup breadcrumbs
- 1 egg
- 2 cloves garlic, minced
- 1/4 cup grated Parmesan cheese
- 1 teaspoon dried oregano
- 1/2 teaspoon salt
- 1/4 teaspoon black pepper
- 8 oz whole wheat spaghetti
- 2 cups marinara sauce
- Fresh parsley, chopped (for garnish)

Instructions:

1. Preheat the oven to 400°F (200°C) and place parchment paper on a baking pan.
2. Combine the ground turkey, breadcrumbs, egg, grated Parmesan cheese, chopped garlic, dried oregano, salt, and black pepper in a big bowl. Blend until well blended.
3. Using the turkey mixture, form meatballs and arrange them on the baking sheet that has been preheated.
4. Bake for 15 to 20 minutes, or until well done, in a preheated oven.
5. Meantime, prepare whole wheat spaghetti according to the directions on the box.
6. In a skillet, warm the marinara sauce over medium heat.

7. Top the cooked whole wheat pasta with chopped fresh parsley and marinara sauce before serving the turkey meatballs.

Nutritional Values (per serving):

Calories: 350
Protein: 25g
Carbohydrates: 30g
Fat: 15g
Potassium: 300mg
Sodium: 400mg
Phosphorus: 250mg

Roasted Vegetable and Quinoa Stuffed Bell Peppers

Preparation Time: 20 minutes
Cooking Time: 35 minutes
Servings: 4

Ingredients:

- 4 large bell peppers, halved and seeds removed
- 1 cup quinoa, cooked
- 2 cups mixed roasted vegetables (such as zucchini, eggplant, bell peppers, cherry tomatoes)
- 1/4 cup crumbled feta cheese
- 2 tablespoons chopped fresh basil
- 2 tablespoons balsamic glaze
- Salt and pepper to taste

Instructions:

1. Adjust the oven temperature to 375°F (190°C) and place parchment paper in a baking dish.
2. Fill the baking dish with the halved bell peppers.
3. Combine cooked quinoa, chopped fresh basil, crumbled feta cheese, mixed

roasted veggies, balsamic glaze, salt, and pepper in a big bowl.
4. Divide the vegetable combination and quinoa among each half of a bell pepper.
5. Bake the baking dish in the preheated oven for 25 to 30 minutes, or until the peppers are soft, covered with aluminum foil.
6. Take off the foil and bake for a further five minutes, or until the tops are browned.
7. Serve hot.

Nutritional Values (per serving):

Calories: 300
Protein: 10g
Carbohydrates: 40g
Fat: 10g
Potassium: 450mg
Sodium: 250mg
Phosphorus: 200mg

Shrimp and Vegetable Skewers with Brown Rice

Preparation Time: 15 *minutes*
Cooking Time: 10 minutes
Servings: 4

Ingredients:

- 1 lb large shrimp, peeled and deveined
- 2 bell peppers, cut into chunks
- 1 zucchini, sliced
- 1 onion, cut into chunks
- 2 tablespoons olive oil
- 2 cloves garlic, minced
- 1 teaspoon smoked paprika

- 1/2 teaspoon cumin
- Salt and pepper to taste
- Cooked brown rice, for serving

Instructions:

1. Turn the heat up to medium-high on the grill or grill pan.
2. Combine the shrimp, bell pepper pieces, zucchini slices, onion chunks, olive oil, minced garlic, cumin, smoked paprika, and salt and pepper in a large bowl and toss until everything is uniformly coated.
3. Thread veggies and prawns onto skewers.
4. Grill the skewers for 3–4 minutes on each side, or until the veggies are soft and the shrimp are pink.
5. Serve hot, accompanied with cooked brown rice.

Nutritional Values (per serving):

Calories: 250
Protein: 20g
Carbohydrates: 20g
Fat: 10g
Potassium: 350mg
Sodium: 300mg
Phosphorus: 200mg

Eggplant Parmesan with Whole Wheat Spaghetti

Preparation Time: 30 minutes
Cooking Time: 40 minutes
Servings: 4

Ingredients:

- 2 large eggplants, sliced into rounds
- 1 cup whole wheat breadcrumbs
- 1/2 cup grated Parmesan cheese

- 2 eggs, beaten
- 2 cups marinara sauce
- 8 oz whole wheat spaghetti
- 1/4 cup chopped fresh basil
- Salt and pepper to taste
- Olive oil for frying

Instructions:

1. Preheat the oven to 375°F (190°C) and place parchment paper on a baking pan.
2. Coat eggplant slices in a combination of whole wheat breadcrumbs, grated Parmesan cheese, salt, and pepper after dipping them into beaten eggs.
3. In a big skillet set over medium-high heat, warm up the olive oil.
4. Add the breaded eggplant slices to the baking sheet that has been prepared after frying them until golden brown on both sides.
5. Bake the eggplant for 15 to 20 minutes in a preheated oven, or until it is soft.
6. Meanwhile, prepare whole wheat pasta as directed on the box.
7. In a saucepan, warm the marinara sauce over medium heat.
8. Arrange roasted eggplant pieces with cooked whole wheat spaghetti, chopped fresh basil, and marinara sauce on top.

Nutritional Values (per serving):

Calories: 350

Protein: 15g

Carbohydrates: 45g

Fat: 10g

Potassium: 400mg

Sodium: 300mg

Phosphorus: 200mg

Beef and Vegetable Stir-Fry with Cauliflower Rice

Preparation Time: 20 minutes
Cooking Time: 15 minutes
Servings: 4

Ingredients:
- 1 lb beef sirloin, thinly sliced
- 2 cups cauliflower rice
- 2 cups mixed vegetables (such as bell peppers, broccoli, carrots, snap peas)
- 2 cloves garlic, minced
- 2 tablespoons low-sodium soy sauce
- 1 tablespoon oyster sauce
- 1 tablespoon sesame oil
- 1 teaspoon grated ginger
- Salt and pepper to taste
- Green onions, chopped (for garnish)

Instructions:
1. In a large skillet or wok, heat the sesame oil over medium-high heat.
2. Stir-fry the grated ginger and minced garlic for 30 seconds.
3. Add the sliced sirloin to the pan and sear it until it becomes brown.
4. Stir-fry the mixed veggies in the pan for five to seven minutes, or until they are crisp-tender.
5. Add the oyster sauce and low-sodium soy sauce, tossing to cover well.
6. Heat the cauliflower rice in a different pan over medium heat until it's well cooked.
7. Top the meat and vegetable stir-fry with chopped green onions and serve it over cauliflower rice.

Nutritional Values (per serving):

Calories: 300
Protein: 25g
Carbohydrates: 15g
Fat: 15g
Potassium: 400mg
Sodium: 350mg
Phosphorus: 250mg

Lentil and Vegetable Soup

Preparation Time: 15 minutes
Cooking Time: 30 minutes
Servings: 6

Ingredients:

- 1 cup dried green lentils, rinsed
- 1 onion, chopped
- 2 carrots, diced
- 2 celery stalks, diced
- 2 cloves garlic, minced
- 1 can (14 oz) diced tomatoes
- 6 cups low-sodium vegetable broth
- 1 teaspoon dried thyme
- 1 teaspoon dried oregano
- Salt and pepper to taste
- Fresh parsley, chopped (for garnish)

Instructions:

1. Rinsed green lentils, diced onion, diced carrots, diced celery, minced garlic, diced tomatoes (with juice), vegetable broth, dried oregano, and thyme should all be combined in a big saucepan.

2. Once the lentils and veggies are soft, bring the soup to a boil, lower the heat, and simmer for 25 to 30 minutes.
3. To taste, add salt and pepper for seasoning.
4. Garnish with freshly cut parsley and serve hot.

Nutritional Values (per serving):

Calories: 200

Protein: 10g

Carbohydrates: 30g

Fat: 5g

Potassium: 400mg

Sodium: 250mg

Phosphorus: 200mg

"I am empowered to make informed decisions about my health and advocate for myself in my healthcare journey".

DESSERTS & SNACKS RECIPES

Fruit Salad with Honey-Lime Dressing

Preparation Time: 15 minutes
Servings: 4

Ingredients:
- 2 cups mixed fresh fruit (such as strawberries, blueberries, grapes, pineapple, kiwi)
- 2 tablespoons honey
- 1 tablespoon lime juice
- Fresh mint leaves for garnish (optional)

Instructions:
1. Clean and cut the fresh fruit mixture into small pieces.
2. To create the dressing, mix the lime juice and honey in a small basin.
3. Drizzle the mixed fruit with the dressing and toss lightly to ensure uniform coating.
4. If preferred, garnish with fresh mint leaves.

Nutritional Values (per serving):
Calories: 80
Protein: 1g
Carbohydrates: 20g
Fat: 0g
Potassium: 150mg
Sodium: 5mg
Phosphorus: 20mg

Dark Chocolate-Dipped Strawberries

Preparation Time: 10 minutes
Cooking Time: 5 minutes
Servings: 4

Ingredients:

- 1 cup dark chocolate chips
- 12 large strawberries

Instructions:

1. Carefully wash and pat dry the strawberries.
2. Melt the dark chocolate chips in 30-second increments in a microwave-safe basin, stirring in between, until smooth.
3. Coat around two-thirds of each strawberry with chocolate by dipping it into the melted confection.
4. Transfer the dipped strawberries to a baking sheet lined with parchment paper and chill until the chocolate solidifies.

Nutritional Values (per serving):

Calories: 120

Protein: 1g

Carbohydrates: 15g

Fat: 7g

Potassium: 150mg

Sodium: 5mg

Phosphorus: 20mg

Greek Yogurt with Fresh Berries and Almonds

Preparation Time: 5 minutes

Servings: 1

Ingredients:
- 1/2 cup Greek yogurt
- 1/2 cup mixed fresh berries (such as strawberries, blueberries, raspberries)
- 1 tablespoon almonds, sliced
- 1 teaspoon honey (optional)

Instructions:
1. Spoon Greek yogurt into a serving bowl.
2. Top with mixed fresh berries and sliced almonds.
3. Drizzle with honey if desired.

Nutritional Values (per serving):

Calories: 150

Protein: 10g

Carbohydrates: 15g

Fat: 7g

Potassium: 200mg

Sodium: 50mg

Phosphorus: 150mg

Baked Apple Slices with Cinnamon

Preparation Time: 10 minutes
Cooking Time: 20 minutes
Servings: 2

Ingredients:

- 2 apples, cored and sliced
- 1 teaspoon cinnamon
- 1 tablespoon honey (optional)

Instructions:

1. Preheat oven to 375°F (190°C) and line a baking sheet with parchment paper.
2. Arrange apple slices on the prepared baking sheet.
3. Sprinkle cinnamon over the apple slices and drizzle with honey if desired.
4. Bake in the preheated oven for 15-20 minutes until apples are tender.

Nutritional Values (per serving):

Calories: 80

Protein: 0g

Carbohydrates: 20g

Fat: 0g

Potassium: 150mg

Sodium: 0mg

Phosphorus: 10mg

Homemade Trail Mix with Nuts, Seeds, and Dried Fruit

Preparation Time: 5 minutes

Servings: 4

Ingredients:
- 1/2 cup almonds
- 1/2 cup walnuts
- 1/4 cup pumpkin seeds
- 1/4 cup dried cranberries
- 1/4 cup dried apricots, chopped

Instructions:
1. In a large bowl, mix together almonds, walnuts, pumpkin seeds, dried cranberries, and chopped dried apricots.
2. Divide the trail mix into individual servings or store in an airtight container for later use.

Nutritional Values (per serving):
Calories: 200

Protein: 5g

Carbohydrates: 15g

Fat: 15g

Potassium: 200mg

Sodium: 0mg

Phosphorus: 100mg

Cottage Cheese with Pineapple and Toasted Coconut

Preparation Time: 5 minutes

Servings: 1

Ingredients:

- 1/2 cup cottage cheese
- 1/2 cup pineapple chunks
- 1 tablespoon toasted coconut flakes

Instructions:

1. Spoon cottage cheese into a serving bowl.
2. Top with pineapple chunks and toasted coconut flakes.

Nutritional Values (per serving):

Calories: 150
Protein: 10g
Carbohydrates: 15g
Fat: 5g
Potassium: 200mg
Sodium: 300mg
Phosphorus: 150mg

Rice Cake with Almond Butter

Preparation Time: 5 minutes

Servings: 1

Ingredients:

- 1 rice cake
- 1 tablespoon almond butter
- Sliced banana (optional)
- Honey (optional)

Instructions:

1. Spread almond butter evenly onto the rice cake.
2. Top with sliced banana and drizzle with honey if desired.

Nutritional Values (per serving):

Calories: 100
Protein: 3g
Carbohydrates: 10g
Fat: 6g
Potassium: 100mg
Sodium: 50mg
Phosphorus: 50mg

Greek Yogurt Bark with Mixed Nuts and Dark Chocolate Chips

Preparation Time: 10 minutes
Freezing Time: 2 hours
Servings: 4

Ingredients:

- 2 cups Greek yogurt
- 1/4 cup mixed nuts, chopped
- 1/4 cup dark chocolate chips

Instructions:

1. Spread parchment paper on a baking sheet.
2. Evenly distribute the Greek yogurt on the parchment paper.
3. Top the Greek yogurt with chopped dark chocolate chips and mixed almonds.
4. Freeze the baking sheet for a minimum of two hours, or until the yogurt solidifies.

5. Once frozen, break the yogurt bark into pieces and serve immediately.

Nutritional Values (per serving):

Calories: 150
Protein: 10g
Carbohydrates: 15g
Fat: 7g
Potassium: 200mg
Sodium: 30mg
Phosphorus: 100mg

Baked Sweet Potato Chips with Sea Salt

Preparation Time: 10 minutes
Cooking Time: 25 minutes
Servings: 4

Ingredients:

- 2 sweet potatoes, thinly sliced
- 2 tablespoons olive oil
- Sea salt to taste

Instructions:

1. Preheat oven to 375°F (190°C) and line a baking sheet with parchment paper.
2. In a large bowl, toss sweet potato slices with olive oil until evenly coated.
3. Arrange sweet potato slices in a single layer on the prepared baking sheet.
4. Sprinkle sea salt over the sweet potato slices.
5. Bake in the preheated oven for 20-25 minutes until chips are crispy and golden brown.

Nutritional Values (per serving):

Calories: 100
Protein: 2g
Carbohydrates: 15g
Fat: 4g
Potassium: 200mg
Sodium: 100mg
Phosphorus: 50mg

SOUP & SALAD RECIPES

Minestrone Soup

Preparation Time: 15 minutes
Cooking Time: 30 minutes
Servings: 6

Ingredients:

- 1 tablespoon olive oil
- 1 onion, diced
- 2 carrots, diced
- 2 celery stalks, diced
- 2 cloves garlic, minced
- 1 can (14 oz) diced tomatoes
- 6 cups vegetable broth
- 1 can (15 oz) kidney beans, drained and rinsed
- 1 cup cooked pasta (such as small shells or elbow macaroni)
- 1 cup chopped spinach or kale
- Salt and pepper to taste
- Grated Parmesan cheese for serving (optional)

Instructions:

1. In a large saucepan over medium heat, warm the olive oil. Add the minced garlic, chopped onion, carrots, and celery. Simmer the veggies for 5 to 7 minutes, or until they are tender.
2. Add the veggie broth and diced tomatoes. Bring to a boil, then simmer for 20 minutes on low heat.
3. Include the cooked pasta, kidney beans, and chopped kale or spinach. Simmer for five more minutes.

4. To taste, add salt and pepper for seasoning. If preferred, top hot servings with grated Parmesan cheese.

Nutritional Values (per serving):

Calories: 200
Protein: 8g
Carbohydrates: 35g
Fat: 3g
Potassium: 500mg
Sodium: 800mg
Phosphorus: 150mg

Chicken Noodle Soup

Preparation Time: 15 minutes
Cooking Time: 30 minutes
Servings: 6

Ingredients:

- 1 tablespoon olive oil
- 1 onion, diced
- 2 carrots, diced
- 2 celery stalks, diced
- 2 cloves garlic, minced
- 6 cups chicken broth
- 2 cups cooked shredded chicken breast
- 1 cup uncooked egg noodles
- 1 teaspoon dried thyme
- Salt and pepper to taste
- Chopped fresh parsley for garnish (optional)

Instructions:

1. In a large saucepan over medium heat, warm the olive oil. Add the minced garlic, chopped onion, carrots, and celery. Simmer the veggies for 5 to 7 minutes, or until they are tender.
2. Add the chicken broth and heat until it boils. Stir in the egg noodles, dry thyme, and shredded chicken. Cook the noodles for 15 minutes by simmering them.
3. To taste, add salt and pepper for seasoning. If preferred, top the hot dish with finely chopped fresh parsley.

Nutritional Values (per serving):

Calories: 250
Protein: 20g
Carbohydrates: 20g
Fat: 8g
Potassium: 400mg
Sodium: 900mg
Phosphorus: 200mg

Butternut Squash Soup

Preparation Time: 15 minutes
Cooking Time: 40 minutes
Servings: 6

Ingredients:

- 1 butternut squash, peeled, seeded, and cubed
- 1 onion, diced
- 2 carrots, diced
- 2 celery stalks, diced
- 2 cloves garlic, minced

- 4 cups vegetable broth
- 1 teaspoon dried sage
- 1/2 teaspoon ground nutmeg
- Salt and pepper to taste
- Coconut milk for serving (optional)

Instructions:

1. Combine chopped onion, carrots, celery, minced garlic, cubed butternut squash, and vegetable broth in a large saucepan.
2. Once the veggies are soft, bring to a boil, lower the heat, and simmer for 30 minutes.
3. Puree the soup with an immersion blender until it's smooth. Alternately, gently transfer the soup to a blender in small batches, purée until smooth, and then pour the soup back into the saucepan.
4. Add the powdered nutmeg and dried sage. To taste, add salt and pepper for seasoning.
5. Present hot, with the option to drizzle with coconut milk.

Nutritional Values (per serving):

Calories: 150

Protein: 3g

Carbohydrates: 30g

Fat: 2g

Potassium: 600mg

Sodium: 700mg

Phosphorus: 100mg

Greek Salad

Preparation Time: 15 minutes
Servings: 4

Ingredients:

- 4 cups chopped romaine lettuce
- 1 cucumber, sliced
- 1 cup cherry tomatoes, halved
- 1/2 red onion, thinly sliced
- 1/4 cup Kalamata olives
- 1/4 cup crumbled feta cheese
- 2 tablespoons olive oil
- 1 tablespoon red wine vinegar
- 1 teaspoon dried oregano
- Salt and pepper to taste

Instructions:

1. Toss together chopped romaine lettuce, cucumber slices, halved cherry tomatoes, thinly sliced red onion, crumbled feta cheese, and Kalamata olives in a big bowl.
2. To create the dressing, combine the olive oil, red wine vinegar, dried oregano, salt, and pepper in a small dish.
3. Drizzle the salad with the dressing and toss to evenly coat.
4. Serve immediately.

Nutritional Values (per serving):

Calories: 120

Protein: 4g

Carbohydrates: 10g

Fat: 7g   Potassium: 300mg

Sodium: 300mg   Phosphorus: 100mg

Caesar Salad

Preparation Time: 10 minutes

Servings: 4

Ingredients:
- 1 head romaine lettuce, chopped
- 1/2 cup Caesar dressing (store-bought or homemade)
- 1/4 cup grated Parmesan cheese
- 1 cup croutons

Instructions:
1. Combine the chopped romaine lettuce and Caesar dressing in a large bowl, tossing to cover the lettuce evenly.
2. Top the salad with grated Parmesan cheese and mix one more.
3. Add croutons on top just before serving.

Nutritional Values (per serving):

Calories: 180

Protein: 5g

Carbohydrates: 15g

Fat: 10g

Potassium: 200mg

Sodium: 300mg

Phosphorus: 100mg

Spinach Salad with Strawberries and Walnuts

Preparation Time: 10 minutes

Servings: 4

Ingredients:

- 4 cups baby spinach leaves
- 1 cup sliced strawberries
- 1/4 cup chopped walnuts
- 2 tablespoons balsamic vinegar
- 1 tablespoon olive oil
- 1 teaspoon honey
- Salt and pepper to taste

Instructions:

1. Combine chopped walnuts, sliced strawberries, and baby spinach leaves in a big basin.
2. To create the dressing, combine the balsamic vinegar, olive oil, honey, salt, and pepper in a small bowl.
3. Drizzle the salad with the dressing and toss to evenly coat.
4. Serve immediately.

Nutritional Values (per serving):

Calories: 100
Protein: 3g
Carbohydrates: 10g
Fat: 6g
Potassium: 300mg
Sodium: 50mg
Phosphorus: 100mg

Quinoa Salad

Preparation Time: 15 minutes
Cooking Time: 15 minutes
Servings: 4

Ingredients:

- 1 cup quinoa, rinsed
- 2 cups water
- 1 cucumber, diced
- 1 bell pepper, diced
- 1/2 red onion, diced
- 1/4 cup chopped fresh parsley
- 1/4 cup crumbled feta cheese
- 2 tablespoons olive oil
- 1 tablespoon lemon juice
- Salt and pepper to taste

Instructions:

1. Boil the water in a medium pot. After the quinoa has been washed, add it, cover it, and simmer it for 15 minutes, or until the water has been absorbed. Take off the heat and let it cool.
2. Put cooked quinoa, diced bell pepper, diced cucumber, diced red onion, chopped fresh parsley, and crumbled feta cheese in a big bowl.
3. To create the dressing, combine the olive oil, lemon juice, salt, and pepper in a small bowl.
4. Drizzle the salad with the dressing and toss to evenly coat.
5. When ready to serve, either serve right away or put in the fridge.

Nutritional Values (per serving):

Calories: 250

Protein: 8g

Carbohydrates: 30g

Fat: 10g

Potassium: 300mg

Sodium: 200mg

Phosphorus: 150mg

Caprese Salad

Preparation Time: 10 minutes
Servings: 4

Ingredients:

- 2 large tomatoes, sliced
- 1 ball fresh mozzarella cheese, sliced
- Fresh basil leaves
- 2 tablespoons balsamic glaze
- Salt and pepper to taste
-

Instructions:

1. Arrange the tomato and mozzarella slices in an alternating fashion on a serving plate.
2. Place a few fresh basil leaves in between the mozzarella and tomato slices.
3. Drizzle the salad with balsamic glaze.
4. To taste, add salt and pepper for seasoning.
5. Serve immediately.

Nutritional Values (per serving):

Calories: 150

Protein: 10g

Carbohydrates: 5g

Fat: 10g

Potassium: 250mg

Sodium: 200mg

Phosphorus: 150mg

"I am grateful for the support of my healthcare team in guiding me on my journey to kidney health".

BEVERAGES

Cucumber Mint Cooler

Preparation Time: 10 minutes

Servings: 2

Ingredients:
- 1 cucumber, peeled and chopped
- 1/4 cup fresh mint leaves
- 2 cups cold water
- Ice cubes
- Optional: Honey or agave syrup for sweetness

Instructions:
1. In a blender, combine chopped cucumber, mint leaves, and cold water.
2. Blend until smooth.
3. Strain the mixture to remove any pulp.
4. Serve over ice cubes.
5. Sweeten with honey or agave syrup if desired.

Nutritional Values (per serving):

Calories: 15

Carbohydrates: 3g

Fiber: 1g

Protein: 1g

Sodium: 2mg

Potassium: 150mg

Berry Blast Smoothie

Preparation Time: 5 minutes
Servings: 2

Ingredients:

- 1 cup mixed berries (strawberries, blueberries, raspberries)
- 1 banana, frozen
- 1 cup unsweetened almond milk
- 1/2 cup Greek yogurt
- 1 tablespoon honey or maple syrup (optional)

Instructions:

1. In a blender, combine mixed berries, frozen banana, almond milk, Greek yogurt, and honey or maple syrup.
2. Blend until smooth.
3. Serve immediately.

Nutritional Values (per serving):

Calories: 150
Carbohydrates: 30g
Fiber: 5g
Protein: 6g
Fat: 2g
Sodium: 100mg
Potassium: 300mg

Watermelon Limeade

Preparation Time: 10 minutes

Servings: 2

Ingredients:

- 2 cups cubed watermelon
- Juice of 2 limes
- 2 cups cold water
- Ice cubes
- Fresh mint leaves for garnish (optional)

Instructions:

1. In a blender, combine cubed watermelon, lime juice, and cold water.
2. Blend until smooth.
3. Strain the mixture to remove any pulp.
4. Serve over ice cubes.
5. Garnish with fresh mint leaves if desired.

Nutritional Values (per serving):

- Calories: 45
- Carbohydrates: 12g
- Fiber: 1g
- Protein: 1g
- Fat: 0g
- Sodium: 2mg
- Potassium: 200mg

Ginger Turmeric Tea

Preparation Time: 15 minutes

Servings: 2

Ingredients:

- 2 cups water
- 1-inch piece of fresh ginger, peeled and thinly sliced
- 1 teaspoon ground turmeric
- 1 tablespoon honey or maple syrup (optional)
- Lemon slices for garnish (optional)

Instructions:

1. In a small saucepan, bring water to a boil.
2. Add sliced ginger and ground turmeric to the boiling water.
3. Reduce heat and simmer for 10 minutes.
4. Strain the tea into cups.
5. Sweeten with honey or maple syrup if desired.
6. Garnish with lemon slices if desired.

Nutritional Values (per serving):

Calories: 10

Carbohydrates: 3g

Fiber: 1g

Sodium: 5mg

Potassium: 50mg

Green Tea Matcha Latte

Preparation Time: 5 minutes
Servings: 2

Ingredients:
- 2 teaspoons matcha green tea powder
- 2 cups unsweetened almond milk
- 1 tablespoon honey or maple syrup (optional)

Instructions:
1. In a small saucepan, heat almond milk over medium heat until hot but not boiling.
2. In a bowl, whisk matcha green tea powder with a small amount of hot almond milk until smooth.
3. Pour the matcha mixture into two cups.
4. Gradually add the remaining hot almond milk to each cup while stirring.
5. Sweeten with honey or maple syrup if desired.

Nutritional Values (per serving):
Calories: 60
Carbohydrates: 6g
Fiber: 1g
Protein: 2g
Fat: 3g
Sodium: 150mg
Potassium: 180mg

"I trust in the healing power of my body and mind, and I believe in my ability to thrive despite any health challenges I may face".

6

KICK START YOUR JOURNEY TO HEALTHIER YOU

Unique Easy to follow 35 Day Meal Plans Tailored for seniors with stage 3 ckd

Day	Breakfast	Lunch	Dinner
1	Veggie Omelette	Lentil Soup	Minestrone Soup
2	Overnight Oats	Greek Salad	Baked Salmon with Lemon
3	Greek Yogurt Parfait	Chicken Stir-Fry	Chicken Noodle Soup
4	Avocado Toast	Vegetable Curry	Lentil Soup
5	Breakfast Burrito	Turkey and Veggie Sandwich	Beef and Vegetable Stir-Fry with Cauliflower Rice
6	Quinoa Breakfast Bowl	Quinoa Salad	Butternut Squash Soup
7	Spinach and Feta Muffins	Shrimp and Veggie Skewers	Eggplant Parmesan

8	Berry Smoothie	Eggplant Parmesan	Greek Salad
9	Cottage Cheese Pancakes	Baked Cod	Lentil Soup
10	Sweet Potato Breakfast Bowl	Black Bean Quesadilla	Chicken Stir-Fry
11	Veggie Omelette	Greek Salad	Quinoa Salad
12	Overnight Oats	Turkey Meatballs	Butternut Squash Soup
13	Greek Yogurt Parfait	Quinoa Salad	Salmon and Avocado Sushi
14	Avocado Toast	Vegetable Stir-Fry	Chicken Noodle Soup
15	Breakfast Burrito	Lentil Soup	Chicken Stir-Fry with Broccoli and Bell Peppers
16	Quinoa Breakfast Bowl	Greek Salad	Butternut Squash Soup
17	Spinach and Feta Muffins	Turkey and Veggie Sandwich	Roasted Vegetable Stuffed Bell Peppers
18	Berry Smoothie	Eggplant Parmesan	Lentil Soup
19	Cottage Cheese Pancakes	Salmon and Avocado Sushi	Chicken Stir-Fry
20	Sweet Potato Breakfast Bowl	Greek Salad	Quinoa Salad
21	Veggie Omelette	Chicken Noodle Soup	Butternut Squash Soup
22	Overnight Oats	Creamy Tomato Soup	Lentil Soup

23	Greek Yogurt Parfait	Quinoa Salad	Roasted Vegetable Stuffed Bell Peppers
24	Avocado Toast	Lentil Soup	Chicken Stir-Fry
25	Breakfast Burrito	Greek Salad	Butternut Squash Soup
26	Quinoa Breakfast Bowl	Vegetable Stir-Fry	Lentil Soup
27	Spinach and Feta Muffins	Turkey Meatballs	Chicken Noodle Soup
28	Berry Smoothie	Quinoa Salad	Creamy Tomato Soup
29	Cottage Cheese Pancakes	Eggplant Parmesan	Butternut Squash Soup
30	Sweet Potato Breakfast Bowl	Chicken Stir-Fry	Lentil Soup
31	Veggie Omelette	Butternut Squash Soup	Quinoa Salad
32	Overnight Oats	Lentil Soup	Turkey Meatballs with Whole Wheat Pasta
33	Greek Yogurt Parfait	Roasted Vegetable Stuffed Bell Peppers	Chicken Noodle Soup
34	Avocado Toast	Quinoa Salad	Butternut Squash Soup
35	Breakfast Burrito	Greek Salad	Lentil Soup

Detailed Comprehensive Grocery Shopping Lists for Convenience

Proteins

Skinless chicken breast

Lean cuts of beef (such as sirloin or tenderloin)

Turkey breast

Fish (salmon, cod, tilapia)

Shellfish (shrimp)

Tofu

Eggs

Cottage cheese

Vegetables

Leafy greens (spinach, kale, lettuce)

Bell peppers

Cucumbers

Tomatoes

Carrots

Broccoli

Cauliflower

Zucchini

Eggplant

Green beans

Onions

Garlic

Fruits

Berries (strawberries, blueberries, raspberries)
Apples
Bananas
Oranges
Watermelon
Pineapple
Grapes
Kiwi
Peaches

Grains

Quinoa
Brown rice
Whole wheat pasta
Whole grain bread
Oats
Barley

Legumes

Lentils
Black beans
Chickpeas
Kidney beans

Dairy and Alternatives

Greek yogurt (unsweetened)

Almond milk (unsweetened)

Soy milk (unsweetened)

Low-fat cheese (such as feta)

Nuts and Seeds

Almonds

Walnuts

Chia seeds

Flaxseeds

Pumpkin seeds

Herbs and Spices

Basil

Parsley

Cilantro

Mint

Dill

Rosemary

Thyme

Oregano

Garlic powder

Onion powder

Ground cumin

Ground coriander

Turmeric

Ginger

Other

Olive oil

Canola oil

Vinegar (balsamic, apple cider)

Honey

Maple syrup

Low-sodium soy sauce

Low-sodium broth (vegetable or chicken)

Tomato paste

Mustard

Low-sodium canned tomatoes

Low-sodium canned beans

Note: When purchasing canned goods, opt for low-sodium or no-sodium varieties whenever possible. Additionally, it's important to read labels carefully and choose products with minimal additives and preservatives. Remember to consult with a healthcare professional or a registered dietitian before making significant changes to your diet, especially if you have stage 3 CKD.

Foods to Eat and Avoid

Foods to Eat

1. Lean protein sources: Skinless chicken, turkey, fish, tofu, eggs.
2. Fresh fruits and vegetables: Berries, apples, cucumbers, carrots, spinach, kale.
3. Whole grains: Quinoa, brown rice, whole wheat pasta, oats.
4. Low-fat dairy or alternatives: Greek yogurt, almond milk, low-fat cheese.
5. Healthy fats: Olive oil, avocado, nuts, seeds.
6. Legumes: Lentils, black beans, chickpeas, kidney beans.
7. Herbs and spices: Basil, parsley, garlic, turmeric, ginger.
8. Limited amounts of potassium-rich fruits and vegetables: Monitor portion sizes of bananas, oranges, potatoes, tomatoes.
9. Limited amounts of phosphorus-rich foods: Monitor portion sizes of dairy, nuts, seeds, whole grains.
10. Plenty of water: Stay hydrated throughout the day.

Foods to Avoid

1. High sodium foods: Processed meats, canned soups, salty snacks.
2. High phosphorus foods: Dairy products, nuts, seeds, whole grains.
3. High potassium foods: Bananas, oranges, potatoes, tomatoes, avocados.
4. Processed and packaged foods: Convenience meals, frozen dinners, packaged snacks.
5. High-fat foods: Fried foods, fatty cuts of meat, full-fat dairy products.
6. Sugary beverages: Soda, sweetened juices, energy drinks.
7. Excessive protein: Limit intake of high protein foods to avoid putting strain on the kidneys.
8. Excessive alcohol: Limit alcohol intake as it can affect kidney function.

9. Caffeine: Limit consumption of caffeinated beverages like coffee and tea.

10. Foods with added phosphates: Processed foods often contain added phosphates, so it's important to read labels carefully.

Accurate Methods Of Using Gram/ounce

Here are the accurate methods of using grams (g) and ounces (oz), as well as how to convert between different measurements:

Using Grams (g) and Ounces (oz):

1. Grams (g):

Grams are a unit of mass commonly used in the metric system.

They are typically used to measure smaller quantities of ingredients, especially in cooking and baking.

A standard metric kitchen scale is often used to accurately measure ingredients in grams.

2. Ounces (oz):

Ounces are a unit of weight commonly used in the imperial system.

In cooking and baking, ounces are often used to measure larger quantities of ingredients, especially in recipes from the United States and some other countries.

There are two main types of ounces: avoirdupois ounces (commonly used for measuring weight) and fluid ounces (used for measuring volume).

Converting Measurements:

1. Converting Grams to Ounces:

To convert grams to ounces, you can use the following conversion factor: 1 ounce = 28.35 grams.

Simply multiply the number of grams by 0.035 to get the equivalent weight in ounces.

2. Converting Ounces to Grams:

To convert ounces to grams, you can use the following conversion factor: 1 gram = 0.035 ounces.

Simply multiply the number of ounces by 28.35 to get the equivalent weight in grams.

Example:

If you have 200 grams of flour and want to convert it to ounces:

200 grams * 0.035 = 7.05 ounces (rounded to two decimal places).

If you have 10 ounces of sugar and want to convert it to grams:

10 ounces * 28.35 = 283.5 grams.

7

LIFESTYLE TIPS

Hydration, Supplements, Exercise, and Stress Management.

For seniors to maintain overall well-being and manage stage 3 CKD, it is important to address issues related to hydration, supplements, exercise, and stress management.

Hydration: Maintaining enough hydrated is crucial for kidney health. To maintain optimal hydration levels without overtaxing their kidneys, seniors with stage 3 CKD should make an effort to consume adequate water. Although there isn't a single, optimal amount of fluid to consume, speaking with a healthcare provider may assist in identifying a person's specific hydration requirements depending on things like renal function and general health.

Supplements: To help meet their nutritional demands, seniors with stage 3 CKD may find it helpful to take certain supplements. But before taking any supplements, it's imperative to speak with a doctor since some of them might damage renal function or interfere with medicine. B vitamins, iron, and vitamin D are a few common supplements for those with chronic kidney disease (CKD).

Exercise: Being physically active regularly is beneficial to general health and may help control CKD symptoms including high blood pressure and weight gain. Moderate exercise according to their skills and health state should be done by seniors with stage 3 CKD. Exercises that enhance cardiovascular health, muscular strength, and general well-being include swimming, walking, and mild strength training.

Stress Management: Prolonged stress may worsen CKD symptoms and have a deleterious effect on renal function. Stress management strategies should be given top priority by seniors with stage 3 CKD to support their mental and emotional health. Techniques like yoga, deep breathing exercises, mindfulness meditation, and time spent in nature may help lower stress levels and enhance the general quality of life.

Why Medical Check-ups

For elders with stage 3 CKD, regular medical examinations are essential to track renal function and general health. During these examinations, blood pressure, urine, and blood tests are used by medical professionals to evaluate renal function. Early identification of renal function abnormalities may lower the risk of consequences including kidney failure and cardiovascular disease as well as assist avoid or halt the course of chronic kidney disease (CKD). Regular examinations also allow medical professionals to modify treatment regimens, prescription drugs, and lifestyle advice as necessary to maximize renal health and general well-being. To guarantee prompt intervention and treatment of their illness, seniors with stage 3 CKD should make frequent follow-up consultations a priority with their healthcare team.

Dinning Out Strategy

For seniors with stage 3 CKD, eating out may be difficult since restaurant food often has high amounts of potassium, phosphorus, and salt, all of which are bad for the kidneys. Dining out may still be fun and kidney-friendly, however, if you prepare ahead and make wise decisions.

1. Do Your Research on Restaurants: Before going out to eat, find out whether establishments are ready to meet particular dietary requirements and provide healthy selections. Seek restaurants that provide customizable food or nutritional information.

2. Make a Plan: Before visiting the restaurant, go over the menu online to find items that are kidney-friendly. In contrast to fried or sautéed foods, choose meals that are baked, steamed, or grilled since these cooking techniques usually need less additional salt and fat.

3. Question Questions: Don't be afraid to question the server about adjustments or replacements of ingredients to make a meal more kidney-friendly. To manage portion sizes and minimize salt consumption, ask for sauces and dressings on the side.

4. Pay Attention to Portion Sizes: Restaurant servings are often greater than required. To prevent overeating and excessive consumption of minerals like potassium and phosphorus, think about splitting a meal with a dining partner or asking for a half quantity.

5. Restrict High-salt Foods: Steer clear of foods like soups, cured meats, and highly seasoned meals that are often high in salt. Select grilled fish or poultry, steaming veggies, and fresh salads with vinaigrette dressing.

6. Make Sensible Drink Selections: Steer clear of sugar-filled beverages and go for water, unsweetened tea, or sparkling water flavored with lime or lemon. Alcohol consumption should be kept to a minimum since it might dehydrate the body and impair renal function.

Seniors with stage 3 CKD may prioritize their renal health and yet enjoy eating out by using these dining out tactics. To preserve ideal kidney function and general well-being, it's critical to make educated decisions, let restaurant employees know about dietary requirements, and watch portion sizes.

CONCLUSION

To sum up, this book "Stage 3 Kidney Disease Diet Cookbook for Seniors" offers a thorough manual for treating stage 3 CKD with wholesome, senior-focused dishes low in potassium, phosphorus, and salt. We've discussed the significance of dietary changes in CKD progression delaying and averting renal failure throughout this book.

We now understand how important it is to maintain kidney health via mindful eating, a balanced diet, and enough water. Every chapter has provided insightful information and useful advice to help seniors confidently manage their nutritional requirements, from comprehending the effects of stage 3 CKD on the elderly to putting methods for eating out and kidney-friendly dishes into everyday meals.

As we come to an end, I urge seniors to embrace the potential of food as medicine and take control of their renal health. Seniors may proactively manage their disease and improve their general well-being by making educated decisions, giving priority to nutrient-rich products, and adopting good eating habits into their daily routine.

Never forget that every meal is a chance to promote kidney function and feed the body. Seniors may take a hopeful and empowering step toward improved kidney health by implementing the advice in this book and collaborating closely with healthcare professionals.

Let's approach the next trip with hope and fortitude. When we band together, we can enable seniors with stage 3 CKD to thrive and lead the greatest possible lives. We hope for a healthy, energetic, and prosperous future.

Dear Reader,

I hope you found value and inspiration in *"Stage 3 Kidney Disease Diet Cookbook for Seniors: Easy-to-Follow Nutritious Low Sodium, Low Phosphorus & Low Potassium Recipes for the Elderly to Manage Stage 3 CKD and Prevent Renal Failure"* We value your feedback!

Please, Could you spare a moment to leave us a review on Amazon? Your review helps other readers discover the book and provides valuable insights for us to improve future editions.

To leave a review simply search for the author Cynthia P Allison on Amazon, click on this book, Scroll down to review this product, click on write a review.

Thank you for your support.

Best regards,

Cynthia P. Allison

"I am resilient and capable of facing any obstacles that come my way with grace and strength".

BONUS

Bonus 1: Free Email Consultation

To have access to the free email consultation, kindly send a message to Cynthia P. Allison at cynthiap.allison@gmail.com for swift response to your question.

Bonus 2: 25 Kidney Health Quiz Questions With Answers for Seniors With Stage 3 Kidney Disease

1. Question: What is the primary function of the kidneys?

2. Question: What is the recommended daily fluid intake for individuals with stage 3 CKD?

3. Question: Which nutrient should be limited in the diet of individuals with stage 3 CKD due to its potential impact on kidney function?

4. Question: What is the term used to describe the buildup of waste products in the blood due to impaired kidney function?

5. Question: Which lifestyle habit is beneficial for kidney health?

6. Question: What is the main source of phosphorus in the diet?

7. Question: Which food group should be limited in a kidney-friendly diet due to its high sodium content?

8. Question: What is the recommended portion size for protein foods in individuals with stage 3 CKD?

9. Question: Which type of beans is lower in potassium: black beans or kidney beans?

10. Question: Which beverage is recommended for maintaining hydration in individuals with stage 3 CKD?

11. Question: What is the role of phosphorus in the body?

12. Question: Which cooking method is preferable for individuals with CKD to reduce sodium intake?

13. Question: What is the main electrolyte that needs to be regulated in individuals with stage 3 CKD?

14. Question: Which fruit is considered high in potassium and should be limited in a kidney-friendly diet?

15. Question: What is the purpose of monitoring blood pressure in individuals with CKD?

16. Question: Which nutrient should be limited in individuals with CKD to prevent bone disease?

17. Question: What is the role of the renal dietitian in managing stage 3 CKD?

18. Question: What is the recommended amount of sodium per day for individuals with CKD?

19. Question: Which type of protein is preferred in a kidney-friendly diet: plant-based or animal-based?

20. Question: What is the purpose of limiting phosphorus intake in individuals with CKD?

21. Question: What is the main function of the glomeruli in the kidneys?

22. Question: Which lifestyle habit can help lower blood pressure and improve kidney function?

23. Question: What is the first sign of kidney damage in individuals with CKD?

24. Question: Which type of bread is lower in phosphorus: white bread or whole wheat bread?

25. Question: What is the purpose of following a low potassium diet in individuals with CKD?

Answers

1. Filtering waste and excess fluids from the blood to form urine.
2. Approximately 6-8 cups of fluids per day, unless otherwise advised by a healthcare provider.

3. Potassium.
4. Uremia.
5. Regular physical activity.
6. Dairy products.
7. Processed foods.
8. Approximately 4-6 ounces per day, divided between meals.
9. Black beans.
10. Water.
11. Phosphorus plays a key role in bone health and energy metabolism.
12. Steaming or baking.
13. Potassium.
14. Bananas.
15. High blood pressure can further damage the kidneys, so it's important to keep it under control.
16. Phosphorus.
17. To provide personalized dietary guidance and support to individuals with CKD.
18. Less than 2,300 milligrams per day.
19. Plant-based protein.
20. To prevent bone disease and mineral imbalances.
21. Filtering waste and excess fluids from the blood.
22. Regular exercise.
23. Protein in the urine (proteinuria).
24. White bread.
25. To prevent hyperkalemia (high potassium levels) and reduce the risk of complications such as irregular heartbeat.

🚀 **Special Offer Just for You! Unlock Exclusive Content!**

Congratulations on choosing *"Stage 3 Kidney Disease Diet Cookbook for Seniors"*! As a valued reader, I have provided exclusive contents to supercharge your renal health journey.

📕 **Explore More Titles by Cynthia P. Allison** 📕

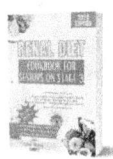

Renal Diet Cookbook for Seniors on Stage 3: A Stage 3 Kidney Disease Diet Handbook with Easy Nutritious Recipes of Low Salt, Low Potassium, and Low Phosphorus Intake. For Easy Access Click 👉 https://rb.gy/sec21v

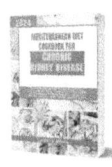

Mediterranean Diet Cookbook for Chronic Kidney Disease: Your Guide to Renal Tasty and Nutritious Recipes, Elevate your well-being through the art of low-sodium, low-phosphorus, low-potassium diets with 14-Days Meal Plan and Easy 5 Mediterranean Friendly Exercises. For Easy Access Click 👉 https://t.ly/aGZs3

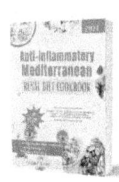

Anti-inflammatory Mediterranean Renal Diet Cookbook: Includes 7-Week Meal Plan with 60+ Nutritious Recipes Specifically Tailored to Fight Inflammation and Boost Kidney Function. For Easy Access Click 👉 https://rb.gy/sy2m3k

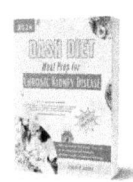
DASH Diet Meal Prep for Chronic Kidney Disease: A Cookbook Guide to Transform Renal Health and Manage Blood Pressure & Cardiovascular Health; Featuring 35-Day Meal Plan & 110+ Kidney-Friendly Recipes. For Easy Access Click 👉 https://rb.gy/k9urej

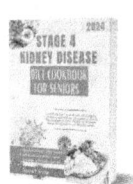
Stage 4 Kidney Disease Diet Cookbook for Seniors: Nutritious Easy-to-Follow Low Sodium, Low Potassium & Low Phosphorus Renal Diet Recipes for the Elderly to Manage Stage 4 CKD & Prevent Renal Failure. For Easy Access Click 👉 https://rb.gy/7wu9fv

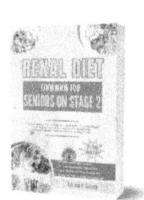
Renal Diet Cookbook for Seniors on Stage 2: A Kidney Disease Diet Handbook with Easy to Follow Recipes of Low Sodium, Low Potassium, & Low Phosphorus Kidney-Friendly Foods for Seniors on Stage 2 CKD. For Easy Access Click 👉 https://rb.gy/mhct0u

❧ Why Choose Cynthia P. Allison?

Expertise: Cynthia P. Allison brings years of experience and expertise to each book.

Practical Wisdom: Every title is packed with actionable advice and real-world insights.

Transformative Impact: Join countless patients and readers who have experienced positive change through Cynthia P. Allison's books and counseling sessions

✺ *Invest in Your Renal Health Improvement Today!* ✺

www.ingramcontent.com/pod-product-compliance
Lightning Source LLC
Chambersburg PA
CBHW082208220526
45470CB00010B/3091